P9-CFA-301

My Secret Mother

My Secret Mother

Two Different Lives, One Heartbreaking Secret

A MEMOIR

Phyllis Whitsell

with Barbara Fisher

Collins

My Secret Mother
Copyright © 2015 by Phyllis Whitsell
All rights reserved.

Published by Collins, an imprint of HarperCollins Publishers Ltd

First published in Great Britain by Mirror Books, an imprint of Trinity Mirror plc, London, under the title *Finding Tipperary Mary*.

First published in Canada in 2016 by Collins in this original trade paperback edition.

No part of this book may be used or reproduced in any manner whatsoever without the prior written permission of the publisher, except in the case of brief quotations embodied in reviews.

HarperCollins books may be purchased for educational, business, or sales promotional use through our Special Markets Department.

HarperCollins Publishers Ltd
2 Bloor Street East, 20th Floor
Toronto, Ontario, Canada
M4W 1A8

www.harpercollins.ca

Library and Archives Canada Cataloguing in Publication information is available upon request.

ISBN 978-1-44345-125-3

Printed and bound in the United States
RRD 9 8 7 6 5 4 3 2 1

Some names have been changed. Every effort has been made to fulfil requirements with regard to reproducing copyright material. The author and publisher will be glad to rectify any omissions at the earliest opportunity.

Contents

Introduction

I only got to know my birth mother when I was 25 years old, but it was some time after her death that I learnt the full details of her early years.

Bridget Mary Larkin was born in Templemore, Co. Tipperary, Ireland, on 11 November 1928. Her immediate family had diminished rather rapidly, and were dysfunctional to say the least. By the age of 14 her mother had died and by 16 she had also lost her father. He'd suffered from ill health for many years; the result of years of smoking and heavy drinking.

According to Bridget he was a 'lazy bastard'. I certainly had the impression that there had been no love lost between her and her father. Forced to grow up quickly, having already left school because of her father's ill health, she was expected to cook and clean the house, do the laundry and look after her little sister Philomena, who was six years younger. Philomena must have only been eight years old when their mother died.

Bridget had no life of her own and did her best to keep the family together. She later told me that she called her daughter Phyllis after her sister Philomena. I was moved that she had given so much thought to choosing my name.

Two of her three brothers had already left the family home when they reached 16. It was as if they were running away from the life they had in Templemore.

Michael, the eldest, who later married and had two daughters, lived in Dublin, and James, known as Jimmie, had lost contact with the family. Bridget often referred to her two older brothers as being decent men who both lived in Dublin, so maybe that is where Jimmie went to live; but it is uncertain what actually happened to him as nobody ever heard from him again. Irish people seem to head for Dublin in the same way as English people head to London to seek their fortune.

Bridget was not allowed to socialise or have any of her own friends. She worked in a factory in Templemore on a part-time basis, and it appears that her life was far from easy. Then Robert, the youngest of the three brothers and a few years older than Bridget, took complete control of my mother and Philomena after the death of their father. When I knew her, she still often talked about drunken men coming back to the house. I was amused when I first heard this, because she was always in such a drunken state herself. I came to realise it was not at all amusing.

I am almost certain that what happened in the house with Robert was the reason why she drank so heavily, from when she was young. If ever she talked about Robert she would go into a rage.

She was always muddled and I often found her difficult to understand but it was clear she was absolutely terrified of him. He was the main reason why she never wanted to go back to Ireland. She would scream and shudder at the mention of his name and stare into space as if she had been hypnotised.

In my heart I always knew something terrible must have happened to her as she appeared so traumatised. I couldn't ask too much, as that was the one thing that she hated more than anything: anyone asking her questions.

She was never prepared to give any information away. But if she had been drinking (which was usually when the truth came out) she would become angry and start shouting, 'He's a wicked man, he just wanted sex,' grinding her teeth with her eyes glazed. If I'm honest she looked like a woman possessed. I realised that whatever had happened to her at the hands of her brother, it was far too painful for her to relive.

Bridget was 22 years old when Keiran was born. After spending three years in a mother-and-baby unit run by nuns, who were extremely strict and cruel, Bridget decided to try and rebuild her life and moved to England. Maybe the shame of having a child out of wedlock was too much for her.

Bridget moved to Coventry in England at the age of 25, desperate to rebuild her life and try to erase what had happened. She'd been forced to leave Keiran with the nuns in Ireland, and she must have felt so lonely and vulnerable. It is not surprising she turned to alcohol; she didn't really stand a chance.

Three years later, on 18 May 1956, she was left holding the baby again. This time that baby was me. There were two versions of who my father was, but the one certain thing is that he was never involved in my life. She coped until I was eight months old, desperately trying to hold on to the one little person she was able to love.

It was now January 1957 and she was a single mother, with little money, living in a cold, damp bedsit. She was becoming increasingly dependent on alcohol. Eventually she made the decision to take me to Father Hudson's Homes, a Catholic adoption society. My mother's previous experiences with nuns had not been good, to say the least, but on my file it had been documented that she had felt the 'strict religious nuns' were 'good at looking after children'.

I knew very little of this when I finally met my mother again, 24 years later, by then she was using her middle name and was known as Tipperary Mary. I had been warned meeting her would have devastating consequences for my family. But, I was still determined to care for her if I could, and I had an idea just how I might do it...

Chapter 1

My Life in the Orphanage

My first childhood memory is of being told off by the strict nuns. If we so much as giggled too loudly we would be told abruptly to be quiet. I always remember them putting their index finger to their lips to reinforce this; the motto at the orphanage was most definitely 'children should be seen and not heard'.

The nursery nurses were very kind, but they were ruled by what the nuns told them to do. The priest visited most mornings and we would be taken into the main hall to say our morning prayers. Sometimes we would go into the church to light a candle. The priest was called Father Taylor and we were all very frightened of him.

The nuns would shout at us when it was time for bed. It was very regimented, and there were no cuddles or bedtime stories. Instead we would have to say the rosary, and as a young child I found it boring.

In the girls' dormitory we had open-plan bays of four beds, with glass panels separating us from the next bay. The priest would often stand by a glass panel watching us get into bed. There was a water font by the door as you walked into the dormitory, and Father Taylor would say in his gruff voice that he had brought the holy water to fill up the font.

When the nuns left the dormitories, we would often have a little jump about on our beds when we thought the coast was clear. I remember having great fun leaping from one bed to the next. Father Taylor often came back into the dormitories. He would just stand watching us jump from one bed to the other, but he never appeared cross with us. He would just say in a deep, rugged Irish voice, putting his finger to his lips as if to imply that it was our little secret, 'Don't tell the sisters or you'll be in trouble.'

In hindsight it was more likely that he would have been in serious trouble for being there in the first place. In 1998, he was imprisoned for sexually abusing young boys (he died in prison in 2001) – as a child I thankfully didn't have any idea that such horrible things could happen. It sent shivers down my spine when I later read about the awful abuse those poor boys had to endure at the hands of that evil man in the 1950s and 1960s.

I did have some happy experiences, and one in particular. When I was about three years old I spent a great deal of time with another orphan called Brendan, who was about five years old. We would say to each other that we hoped one day we would be able to be brother and sister.

I can honestly say that Brendan was the first person in my young life that I'd had such strong feelings for, and that is why he made such a lasting impression. For a lot of children their mother or father would be that person, and their feelings would be there automatically; it would be so natural they wouldn't even give it a second thought. But often, as an adopted child, your memories are much more vivid.

Sometimes the children would be taken out by the nursery nurses to the post office in the village. We would all be so excited. It was as if we were going on our holidays. Other shoppers stopped us in the street and asked, 'Are you the children from the orphanage?' The nursery nurses would politely nod their heads and smile.

If we were good the nursery nurses would buy us

some sweets to share, and I would always share my sweets with Brendan. There was a busy road to cross, so we were told by the nursery nurses to find a partner, hold each other's hands and walk in a crocodile. Inevitably Brendan would be holding my hand. He always seemed to want to protect me, he'd say, 'I am looking after my little sister so she doesn't get hurt.'

Brendan would often look sad and I would put my arm around him and ask, 'Why are you upset?' He would look at me and say, 'All I want is a mummy and daddy and you as my little sister.' He was so young himself, but acted so grown up. He would say, 'I am going to be your big brother and nobody is going to touch my little sister.' Now I look back and hope that he was not hurt in any way, as he often seemed so upset.

We'd play together for hours, me in my little bossy way, but he never seemed to mind. We just enjoyed spending time together doing normal things that children do. We were so happy playing our pretend games, lost in our own little world. I can truly say we shared a special bond.

Eventually a couple who wanted to adopt a little boy was found for Brendan. He was nearly six years old by then. The couple had no children of their own so Brendan not surprisingly asked the nuns, 'Can Phyllis come with me and be my little sister please?', exaggerating his 'pleeeaase' while desperately hoping they would say yes.

He put his hands together as if he was praying for it to happen. But the nuns replied in their usual stern, dismissive voices, 'NO!' By now he was jumping up and down excitedly, tugging at their long white habits, which would have annoyed them, and the answer remained unchanged.

I was never going to be Brendan's little sister. The only brother I wanted was Brendan, but that was not going to happen.

The day I was dreading eventually arrived, just before Christmas time, and I would never see Brendan again. It was one of the saddest times of my life. I really felt that I had lost my big brother, who looked after me and made me feel safe. We cried our hearts out and promised each other that one day we would run away together, but we both knew really that it would never happen.

Brendan packed a small suitcase and I gave him my favourite toy as a keepsake, so that he could hold it at night when he was lonely and dream of his little sister. I remember the nuns asking me if I was sure that I wanted to give Brendan my favourite cuddly toy. It was the teddy bear I'd had as a baby, the one my mother left for me, but I wanted to give him something that was very precious, just like he was. Yes, they were right, I would be crying, but it would be for Brendan and not my teddy bear.

Standing on the steps of the orphanage I gave Brendan a kiss and a cuddle, and we were both crying. Eventually Brendan's new mother took charge and managed to get him into the car. I waved Brendan goodbye, holding Sister Theresa's hand. I watched him sitting in the car with tears running down his face and such a sad smile. Then he was suddenly kneeling and looking out of the back of the car window, pretending that the teddy bear was also waving. I remember the nun tightly squeezing my little hand so hard that it hurt; but not as much as I was hurting inside. Sister Theresa was very kind to me. I think she realised how upset I was and told me not to cry as very soon I would be 'special' too and have a new mummy and daddy, and maybe even brothers and sisters of my own.

All I wanted was to have Brendan back. The car that

was taking him away drove slowly down the path and was very quickly hidden by the large green oak trees that stood tall at the end of the drive. I kept thinking about Brendan having his first Christmas with his new parents. Sister Theresa was my favourite nun. Later I asked her whether she thought Father Christmas could work his magic and let Brendan have me as his little sister for Christmas. She laughed at my impossible request and hugged me, which I so needed. She told me things would improve, although I didn't think I would ever feel better.

She took me into the kitchen, which was usually out of bounds for the children. She sat me on the stainless steel work surface which felt cold on the back of my legs. I would normally have been so excited. I was even given a hot homemade cake which I had never had before. But nothing was going to stop me from missing Brendan and hurting inside.

I loved Brendan in a way you love your brother or sister, and he was the closest thing I'd had to family. Those feelings are very precious and priceless but often just taken for granted until you lose that person. Then you feel a terrible loss, an emptiness inside your stomach that is so unbearable that it hurts.

Father Taylor came into the main entrance and after speaking to Sister Theresa he took my hand and led me into the church. He suggested that we light a candle for Brendan and his new parents. He was standing at the altar looking down at me alone in the front pew. Every so often I had a little whimper to myself. We said a short prayer for Brendan but it gave me no comfort.

In time things went back to the usual routine but I never forgot Brendan and I do hope he had a happy childhood. Maybe he did have a little sister; if not, at least he had my teddy bear to cuddle at night. He may have children of his own now, even grandchildren. I would love to meet up with him again as he had such an impact on my life.

The nuns at the orphanage had always told me that I needed to be part of a family unit, as I was a chatterbox and enjoyed other children's company. So when Mr and Mrs Price first made enquiries about adopting a little girl, I was the obvious choice. They already had three children of their own: two boys, Kevin aged twelve and Anthony aged nine and their 'delicate' daughter Carole who was five years old.

Mr and Mrs Price ticked all the right boxes. They

were supposedly happily married and a good Catholic family. My adoptive mother had a difficult pregnancy with Carole and apparently was advised by the medical profession not to have any more children of her own, so adopting a child seemed the obvious choice. To give a home to a child from the Catholic orphanage in Coleshill, Birmingham, was seen as a respectable thing to do amongst the church community. I remember hearing comments like 'you must be a good Catholic if you want to adopt a child'.

I was first introduced to my new family in February 1960, when I was nearly four years old. It was a Saturday afternoon and I was dressed up for the occasion; a dress I usually wore on Sundays to go to church and a ribbon in my hair. I was taken into the main office to see Sister Bernadette, the Mother Superior, and I knew it must be something serious.

Sister Theresa was holding my hand to give me some much needed moral support. She knelt down to whisper in my ear, 'This might be your new mummy and daddy.' I remember even at such a young age having butterflies in my stomach and feeling like running in the opposite direction. Sister Theresa gently squeezed my hand and gave me a comforting smile. She reassured me, saying, 'Don't worry, it's just to have a little chat and get to know each other.'

The big wooden door was opened very slowly by Sister Theresa. It made a loud squeaking noise. I took a deep breath and just walked into the office. I could feel my entire body shaking, but for the only time I can recall, Mother Superior was smiling at me. Sitting behind her big wooden polished desk with her hands together, she introduced me to my new mother and father, saying, 'They are looking for a little sister for their own daughter.'

Those words stayed with me for such a long time. I asked, 'Can't I be their daughter too?' They all just laughed. They had no idea how hurt I was feeling inside by such an insensitive comment. I wanted a mother and father, and maybe brothers and sisters, but I didn't want to be a little sister for their daughter.

The only person I wanted to be a little sister to was Brendan, and that was never going to happen. I felt as if they were coming to buy me from a toy shop, just like a new doll. 'We want a baby sister for our daughter please.' Well, at least that is how it made me feel.

My new father got out of his chair and bent down so he was at my level, which did help me feel less anxious.

He gave me a lovely smile, which I will always remember, and took my now sweaty little hand from Sister Theresa's grasp and said, 'Hello Phyllis, I hope I can be your new daddy.'

I was now starting to feel more relaxed. He poured me a drink of orange squash from a specially prepared tray. I remember sipping the drink very slowly, almost trying to hide behind the glass. The lady stayed in her seat and just looked me up and down. She looked so cross, and I was not impressed with my new mother in the slightest. It was as if she was putting on an act trying to be 'posh', which I later discovered was what she always did when she was around people she didn't know. This was especially if she thought they were important and I'm inclined to think that Mother Superior would have been on her 'important list'.

After the first meeting, I remember Canon Flynn asking if I liked my new parents. This surprised me, and I replied, 'I like my daddy but my mummy looked cross.' I am sure to this day that my opinion didn't make the slightest bit of difference as nothing else was ever said. They had found a good Catholic family, I would have siblings – in theory it should work.

The next Sunday they came to visit me again, and this time they brought Carole with them. She had brown curly hair so we looked nothing like sisters as I had straight blonde hair. She was shy at first but did seem a little excited to meet me. We walked into the grounds of the orphanage and played on the swings and slides. My new father pushed me on the swings and I remember calling him Daddy for the very first time. 'Push me higher, Daddy!' I shouted. It was lovely and sunny, and I felt so happy. I remember enjoying the day and thinking to myself how lovely it was to have someone to visit me. I would have something to look forward to at the weekends.

Chapter 2

Family Life

The following week could not come quickly enough and it was then that I met my two brothers, Anthony and Kevin. I was so excited. I remember asking Sister Theresa, 'How long will it be until they are here?'

She told me to go upstairs and look out of the bay window, as it overlooked the car park. I would be able to see them all arriving. It was probably only about half an hour, but for a little girl waiting to meet her new family it was an eternity.

As I saw them walking across the drive I ran downstairs excitedly to meet them all. Sister Theresa held my hand and opened the big wooden double doors at the entrance to the orphanage.

Again it was a lovely sunny day, and I was so full of anticipation at meeting my whole family that I had a funny feeling in my stomach. Sister Theresa had allowed me to miss breakfast as she knew I was feeling nervous at the thought of meeting them. She was so kind to me and stayed close to give me much-needed moral support.

The man who was to be my new father gave me a really tight hug. Even now, as I think of that embrace, I have a wonderful warm feeling inside.

Anthony was walking in front and looked really grumpy, and certainly not too impressed about having a new little sister. I suppose that, as a ten-year-old boy, he would rather have been playing with his friends and climbing trees. Kevin was 13 and appeared much happier, he gave me a big smile. He actually seemed quite happy at the prospect of having a new little sister.

My new mother was anything but happy and stood stern-faced, holding Carole's hand. Carole stood shyly behind her mother as if she did not want any contact with me at all. I did manage to get a glimpse of her face – to me, she seemed to be thinking, This is my mummy and I am not going to share her with you.

I felt like an outsider. All I wanted was for this lady to give some kind of gesture to show that she cared; just a smile or a small embrace would have helped me feel more relaxed and part of this family.

I was taken with my prospective siblings to play together in the grounds of the orphanage. Kevin took me by the hand and we both ran to the lake. Normally we children would not be allowed to go that far, but as I was with my potential new family I am sure that Sister Theresa felt that I was safe. She went back into the orphanage and left us to it.

Kevin excitedly showed me the tadpoles in the lake, and told me they would eventually turn into frogs. I remember feeling very happy. Despite the fact that my new mother, sister and other brother Anthony were not what I had hoped for, I liked my new father and brother Kevin. For a little girl of four desperate to have a family of her own, it was enough for now.

The Prices visited me several times, usually on Sundays. I always enjoyed their visits, even though my new mother never really made me feel she was happy to have me as her daughter. I was aware at the time that she seemed more concerned about Carole accepting me as her sister. I was confused because my adoptive mother was constantly saying that Carole was so pleased to be having a new sister, but to me it seemed as if that was the last thing she wanted.

***

One weekend I visited them at their house. I was very excited as I packed a small bag for the overnight stay in a proper family home. Not surprisingly, it was my new father and big brother Kevin who picked me up and took me to their house. We travelled on two buses, which seemed to take ages. I couldn't remember ever travelling on a bus before. Although not the complete unit I had hoped for, for the first time in my short life I felt like part of a family and I felt that someone cared about me. We stopped on the way and Kevin bought me an ice cream. Perhaps things were going to be all right after all.

When we arrived at the house, Kevin played in the garden with me, swinging me round and round. I was so dizzy I eventually fell over and grazed my knee. Mum shouted at him, 'We might not be able to keep Phyllis now because of what you have done.' That worried me for days, and when I returned to the orphanage I did my best to hide my knee from the nuns. They never noticed, so I was worrying about nothing. I was growing up and it was becoming more difficult to find a suitable family prepared to adopt me, so a small graze on my knee was not going to stop that happening.

***

The one person I was going to miss from the orphanage was my favourite nun, Sister Theresa. She helped me pack my few belongings in a small suitcase the night before I left. I remember sobbing my little heart out and tears running down my face.

She pulled a small handkerchief from the pocket of her long white habit and my tears halted as I noticed my name had been embroidered in the corner. Sister Theresa wiped my face with this very special handkerchief and gave me a loving cuddle.

'Don't cry, you will soon be with your new family and everything will be just fine,' she said. She told me that she would pray that I would have a happy childhood.

She neatly folded the handkerchief she had given to me, which by now was damp with my tears, and put it inside my bag so that I would be able to take it to my new home for a keepsake, in memory of my beloved Sister Theresa. I never did see her again, but I kept the handkerchief under my pillow as I went to sleep at night.

By the end of July 1960 I had moved in with my new family, and at first it was very exciting. I was to share the back bedroom with Carole, and we both eagerly ran upstairs.

Carole quickly jumped onto her bed, which was by the window. There was a selection of dolls and teddies on her bed. My adoptive mother immediately pointed to the other bed, and as I looked over I noticed a new doll sitting there. Without thinking I commented, 'I've only got one doll.' I'm sure I was just feeling a little insecure in my new environment, but I was told sharply, 'Your sister is older than you so she will always have more than you.' I suppose I sounded like a spoilt little girl, they had bought me a brand new doll, but I had been made to feel different immediately.

It was the next morning when I first saw my adoptive mother's angry face. In the orphanage we often jumped on each other's bed. So that first morning I jumped on my sister's bed, feeling so happy. I looked out of the window and noticed my new mummy hanging washing on the line. I gently waved and smiled. I was finally going to be part of a real family. But her face changed and looked so cross as she shouted, 'I hope you haven't woken Carole up, get off her bed immediately.' I hoped she wasn't always going to be shouting at me like that.

My adoptive father was very kind. He baked a cake,

and I sat on a stool in the kitchen waiting for it to cool down so I could help him put the icing on the top. He laughed at my impatience and told me it would be a few hours before I could put the icing on.

They lived in a three-bedroom, semi-detached house in a cul de sac. All the houses looked the same, with white render on the outside walls, so different from the darker bricks of the orphanage. The house was between two parks, it had a fairly big front garden (and a lovely big back garden) and directly across the road there was a grass play area with an embankment and a stream.

It was a wonderful setting for me to explore in my first few days, under the watchful eye of my adoptive father, with whom I quickly formed a special bond. Dad retrieved an old fishing net from his cramped shed, and my face lit up when I saw the old jam jar he lifted up so gently, as he removed a large cobweb from around the rim. In the stream there were pebbles that looked as if they'd been polished by the clear water. As I watched the fishes swimming between those pebbles I felt the warmth of the sun on my back. I had never done anything like this before.

We didn't actually catch any fish on that particular day but I had such fun. Despite holding my father's hand tightly I lost his grip and slipped on one of those wet pebbles. My socks and sandals were soaking wet.

Mum shouted at him for not watching what I was doing, 'She will catch her death of cold!' I'd only been there a day and I hoped I would live to see another day with the Price family. I very quickly realised that she was the boss of the household.

While I felt happy to be part of a new family, I also felt confused by my adoptive mother's behaviour. She seemed annoyed if I ever mentioned the time I had spent at the orphanage. It was as if I was expected to erase over four years of my childhood from my memory. I hoped things would improve and they would eventually love me as their daughter.

Ten days after arriving, my new parents packed to go to Ireland, and I was thrilled to be going with them! We travelled to Holyhead by train and then took a boat. Even now I find it so exciting travelling on boats; it is a feeling that has always stayed with me. I remember asking my dad, 'Will I be able to put my hand in the sea?' – which obviously caused great laughter at my naivety.

I had little experience of anything other than being in an orphanage but now I had a whole new extended family to meet: uncles, aunts and lots of cousins who were very welcoming. It was the first time I felt like part of the family.

But my new mother was just putting on a show for her family and friends in Ireland, and treated me differently behind closed doors. When I was in the garden with my cousins, my Auntie Betty said, 'How lovely that you have two big brothers and a sister.' I had been told not to say anything about the orphanage, but I forgot and said, 'I had Brendan, he was going to be my big brother and look after me, but he has a new mummy and daddy.'

Mum took me to one side, 'Please don't say anything about that. How would it make Kevin and Anthony feel – they're your brothers now.'

When no one was around, she went into great detail about how I should be grateful because they had taken me out of the orphanage. She said, 'If it wasn't for us you would still be in the orphanage and would have spent all your childhood there. I bet people think I want my head looking at, taking on another child, when I already have three children of my own. I suppose I will get my reward in heaven.' Her cruel words upset me. Instead of letting me have any settling-in time she isolated me from the family, and didn't seem to think of my feelings.

I was meant to start school in September, but my mother didn't want me to go to a non-Catholic school so I stayed at home for a few months in limbo. She said, 'We will wait until January as there is a new Catholic school opening and it is closer to where we live.' I actually found myself missing the company of the children in the orphanage.

I asked why I couldn't go to the same school as my brothers and sister but Mum just shouted at me, 'No, that will not happen. People will ask too many questions. Do you want everyone to know you are adopted? You will be different to everyone else. It must be kept a secret. Our family secret. Forget about being adopted, you are now part of this family. Do you want everyone to know you were an orphan?' But already I felt anything but part of that family, and now I felt ashamed that I had been adopted.

My mother and I would go on the bus to pick up Carole and Anthony from school. Kevin was at secondary school and was allowed to go home by himself.

Mum would always start talking to someone, and they would ask, 'Why is your little girl not at school today? Is she poorly?' At first I was keen to go on a bus ride, but now I started to dread them. My mother would say, 'If anyone asks you your age tell them you are three-and-a-half years old, and then they will not keep asking me why you are not at school.'

She would do her best to start up a conversation with anyone who was prepared to listen. I always felt very nervous about what questions they'd ask. I often thought to myself, Why can't she just have a chat with me? One bus journey I remember well. She started chatting to a woman also on her way to pick up her children from school. The woman said to my mother, 'Are you looking after this little girl for your friend?'

Mum replied, 'No, this is my daughter.'

The woman looked surprised and said, 'But she looks nothing like your other children.'

I turned to look out of the window, as by now I was feeling sick and worried about her next question and almost dreading my mother's reply. I heard her whisper to the woman, as she thought I was not listening, 'We adopted her from Father Hudson's Homes, as Carole wanted a little sister.'

I was hurting so much inside. I felt angry and upset at the same time. Why was I not allowed to tell anyone about my adoption, yet she could tell this woman everything, even though she hardly knew her?

My feelings didn't seem to matter. If she needed to remove something from my face, she'd rub fiercely with a spit dampened handkerchief. Carol's face would be gently wiped, because she was the delicate one. When my mother got angry her whole face changed and she would stare at me for a long time. This was something she didn't seem to do to her natural children, or at least if she did I never noticed. I think the angry face was saved just for me, and it terrified me. Yes, she did tell her own children off, but the real anger did not seem to be there.

Perhaps she was worried about the type of person I would turn out to be. Although I knew nothing about my birth mother, of course my adoptive mother would have been told about her drinking and lack of a husband. Maybe she thought some of her traits would come out in me. She may have worried that I would become out of control, that some of my real mother's 'bad blood' would somehow be passed on to me.

In hindsight, I believe this is the main reason why she was so strict with me. At the time, I just felt like the cuckoo in the nest. I often thought about the two people who meant the most to me, Brendan and Sister Theresa, and wished I could tell them how much I was hurting inside.

In November a school inspector had visited the house and asked my mother, 'Why has Phyllis not started school yet?' Mum explained that she was waiting for the new Catholic school to open but that would be a few more months. The inspector said that I needed to be educated as soon as possible, and the school around the corner had a vacancy. I was to start the following Monday.

My mother was horrified at the thought of having to take me to a Church of England school. She made me feel as if I was about to go in front of a firing squad; as if I were going somewhere terrible.

Most children are a little bit worried about their first day at school and hope they will make new friends – their mothers usually reassure them that they don't need to worry and they will be fine. I was petrified, and was actually told not to make any friends.

***

When I started it was almost Christmas and the end of term so I only went to that school for three weeks, but it seemed a hell of a lot longer. I hated every minute.

Every day when my mother picked me up she would make it clear that I should not be at a Church of England school. 'It is not where you belong,' she would tell me. 'They are not the same type of people as us.' I didn't understand what she meant, so it just made me feel very scared, as if I was going to be damaged in some way by mixing with non-Catholic people. This affected me for a long time and I would worry about talking to people in case they were not Catholics.

My mother always thought she was right; my poor father just went along with whatever she said. I suppose he did it for a quiet life. She was most certainly the boss and made all the decisions which were to affect me.

By January 1961 the new school had been built and was ready for all the children to start there at the beginning of the term. This time it was going to be exciting. Carole was also starting at the same school and for once she treated me like her little sister; she actually seemed quite protective towards me.

We put on our new school uniforms. I remember wearing a grey pinafore which had a small zip at the front. It was something that Carole had grown out of but that didn't bother me. At least my nice red tie was new, and I had a new pair of shiny shoes, so it wasn't so bad.

I decided to put my very special handkerchief that Sister Theresa had given me in my zipped pocket. As the handkerchief had my name on it, I could show it to the teachers if they forgot my name. Then they would know I was Phyllis. It also made me feel close to Sister Theresa, which was lovely.

Anyway, we set out for our first day at school. I was holding Carole's hand and we skipped happily as we went along singing a nursery song. ('This is the way we wash our clothes, wash our clothes, wash our clothes; this is the way we wash our clothes on a cold and frosty morning.') It was one of the nicest feelings I can ever recall having as a young child. I felt like I belonged to a family and I was so happy.

We walked across the park to get to the school, which was called St Margaret Mary's. I was thinking to myself that at least I will be allowed to make some new friends because they will also be Catholics, which made me really happy.

Kevin and Anthony had by now started secondary school, and our mother was trying to hide her age. Carole and I were told, 'Don't say you have any older brothers as I don't want the school to know how old I am.' Yet another secret I had to keep to myself. It never seemed to bother Carole, but I suppose she wasn't a chatterbox like me so perhaps keeping secrets wasn't so hard for her.

We had to report to the school office, and our mother held our hands, telling us to be quiet while she spoke to the headmaster, Mr O'Laughlin. Everything seemed so perfect, so normal for a short time, but I'm afraid to say that was to be short-lived.

Mr O' Laughlin was a very tall man. He asked my mother her daughters' names, so he could check which class we would be in. My mother started to whisper her reply, forcing the headmaster to bend down so he was in earshot, 'Carole, who is our own daughter, and Phyllis, who we adopted from Father Hudson's Homes; but it is best if no one else knows that Phyllis is adopted.'

This immediately made me feel different from all the other children, as if being adopted was something so bad that you should be ashamed of it and nobody should ever know. My mother continued, 'Phyllis is not a name we would have picked for our own daughter as it does not really go with our surname. Phyllis was only given one name, poor thing, but I suppose we will get used to it.'

Mr O'Laughlin seemed uneasy with my mother's long explanation. He said, 'I think it's a lovely name.' I told him about my special handkerchief that had my name on it which I could show my teacher, to remind her of my name if she forgot it. He laughed and said I was the only Phyllis in the school, he was sure they would not forget 'such a lovely name'. He was very kind and gave me a reassuring pat on the head.

With all the confusion I somehow ended up in the wrong classroom. By now all the parents had left and there was a lot of organising to be done by the teachers. I spent the whole morning in Carole's class but by lunchtime a teacher came into the classroom and said, 'I think there is a little girl in the wrong class and her name is Phyllis.' I started to cry as I was sure I would be told off for not listening to what class I should have been in, but she just smiled and took my hand and told me not to worry. I told her I wanted to stay with my sister, she smiled again and said, 'You are too young to be in this class, but you can play with your sister later.'

I ran eagerly over to Carole in the playground in the afternoon, but by now she had made a new friend called Kathleen and I think she was becoming tired of looking after her little sister. I didn't make any friends myself that day; I was still thinking about how I felt at the first school, and how making friends had not been such an easy thing to do. Also, I now didn't relish the thought of having to tell anyone my name in case they made fun of me. I was starting to hate my name, and thought, I wish I was called something else. I even thought of pretending that I was called Brenda, as it reminded me of Brendan, but I knew Carole would have told everyone that I was telling lies and I was sure to be told off for embarrassing her.

Instead I ran around the playground on my own. It was a really windy afternoon so I thought it would be great fun to play with my special handkerchief and remember Sister Theresa and how kind she had always been to me. That would make me feel happy and not so lonely in such a big playground. That lovely comforting feeling did not last for long.

Suddenly there was a great gust of wind and, as I was spinning around, the handkerchief escaped from my grasp and blew away. I ran frantically to try and retrieve it, but the more I ran the quicker it flew. I was so distracted and desperate to find it that I didn't hear the school bell for the end of playtime.

The bell would ring once and all the children had to stand perfectly still like statues, not moving a muscle. It would not be rung again until all the children were perfectly still, and there was I running frantically around the playground crying and trying to chase my hankie, which was blowing further and further away. All the children were laughing at me running around like a naughty little girl. I knew I was in trouble by the look on the teacher's face as she shouted at me to get to the front of the queue.

By now I was inconsolable. I had lost the handkerchief that I held at night to help me to go to sleep, that wiped away my tears when I cried, which still smelled of Sister Theresa; and which had gone forever. I will never forget the feeling of emptiness I had. But I feared that, if I had told anyone, they would laugh their heads off for making such a great fuss about a silly hankie.

As the weeks went by I soon settled well into my new school and started to make friends. I always felt sad when I thought of the very special handkerchief I had lost, and would often walk around the playground in the hope that I might be lucky enough to find it again in the long grass. But it had blown away, never to be seen again.

One friend I felt particularly close to was Pauline. We would walk around the playground holding hands, as children do, and say to each other we were best friends. Pauline would often say that, as best friends, you should tell each other all your secrets. Looking back now I think she knew I was adopted, as our mothers would regularly be chatting at the school gate, and I am sure Pauline's mum would have been told, in a whisper, about my adoption.

Pauline would often say, 'You look nothing like your sister. Are you sure you really are sisters?' But I had been told by my mother that under no circumstances must I ever tell anyone that I had been adopted.

Eventually I decided to tell Pauline, stressing that she must never tell anyone. For a few days I felt happy and relieved that I had shared my special secret with my best friend. But children invariably fall out from time to time, and sure enough we had our first squabble, no doubt about something trivial. I don't really remember, but what I do remember was that we were no longer best friends and she made my time at school hell.

She started to blackmail me. I would have to give her things, like a packet of crisps or my favourite hair band, which I would later be told off for losing. If I didn't give her what she wanted she would threaten to tell the whole school that I was adopted, and that was the last thing I ever wanted to happen and she knew it. I remember dreading assembly at school, as I always imagined Pauline marching to the front of the hall and announcing, 'Phyllis is adopted, you know.' I would even have nightmares about it, but thankfully it never did happen.

Children can be so cruel, and she was a proper bully. It was so wrong and at the time I thought I had nobody I could confide in. When I went to bed at night I often cried myself to sleep wishing I had my special handkerchief from Sister Theresa to wipe away my tears, or Brendan as my big brother to tell her to leave me alone.

I decided that my mother must have been right. Being adopted should be kept a secret and was something to be ashamed of. I certainly knew I would never be able to confide in my mother and tell her how Pauline had treated me. As she always told me never to tell a soul, I knew I would have been in so much trouble for being disobedient. So for the rest of my childhood

I kept this secret to myself to ensure that I didn't have to go through such a dreadful experience again. I never did tell another soul until I got married years later.

Thankfully the bullying did eventually stop, and if any of the children knew about my adoption they never mentioned it to me. By the time I went back to school after the summer break I was in a new school year, and there was now a new reception class, so I was feeling quite grown up, as you do when the younger children arrive and suddenly you are not one of the smallest in the school. I was actually starting to enjoy school and was happy with that part of my life; it was so much better than the previous year.

The same could not be said for my family life. I felt very detached from them, and certainly did not feel as if I belonged to a loving and secure family. Carole often made me feel as though she resented having me as her sister. I sometimes thought she felt it made her life harder by having me around. Financially it was often a struggle, so maybe she felt that because I was now part of the family she had to go without things.

I had been told about their holiday in Skegness the

year before I was adopted. One day Carole had walked along the pier when it was extremely windy, and this had made her hair curly and had left her very anxious, which caused her to have 'sugar diabetes'. This was the reason she was so delicate and, at the time, I understood why she was given more attention. When I found out years later that she had never been diabetic it proved to me how far my mother was prepared to go in order to justify showing more kindness to Carole than me. The reason Carole had all the treats, even having lots of sweets, was that she was their own daughter and I was adopted.

Carole always seemed to be telling tales, hoping to get me into some kind of trouble. She would often scream at the top of her voice, 'Phyllis has just pinched my arm for no reason.' I used to think to myself, If I had a reason for pinching your arm would that somehow make it right? Of course it wouldn't, but often the things Carole said never seemed to make sense, certainly not to me. I think she knew if she cried loudly enough I would get into trouble. My adoptive mother was never prepared to listen to my side of the story; the fact that Carole was crying was enough for her to believe that I had done something wrong and been cruel in some way to her fragile daughter. I would be reprimanded sternly, 'You know she is delicate.'

Nobody else seemed to see through Carole's crocodile tears, which at the time was so frustrating. She appeared to fool the whole family and was more than happy with that.

I now realise that my mother was so close-minded that I would never have been able to communicate with her. She believed that what she said and did was always right and was never prepared to listen to other people's points of view. Well, certainly not her adopted daughter's.

As a little girl I didn't stand a chance of explaining to her how I was feeling, or for her to have listened, understood and actually acted upon it. I was the adopted daughter and was always going to be treated as a child they had from the orphanage, not a child that they had conceived together: their natural child.

Sometimes my father tried to treat me in a loving way, as a father should treat his daughter. He would give me an extra hug, which, strangely enough, was never in the presence of my mother. On one occasion when we were sitting in the lounge, the door started to open. Dad was just lifting his arm up to give me a cuddle, but then suddenly he pulled away. As it happens it was only our pet dog, who had managed to open the door with her little wet nose.

I did wonder why my father was so nervous of showing me any affection whenever my mother was about, and realised that it was not normal because of things I heard other children say. I would feel upset and sometimes even angry that he was not allowed to show me the slightest bit of affection in case Carole got jealous. It was just so unfair. He would tell me not to worry, 'you know we love you as much as her'. But this just made me feel worse as he would never have pulled his arm away from Carole if he was about to give her a cuddle. She could have all the cuddles in the world, which is how it should be.

My adoption was always at the front of my mind because my adoptive mother never seemed to go one day without mentioning it. But my parents never seemed to realise that I noticed that I was treated differently from their own daughter, and how unloved I often felt. I think in their minds they honestly believed they were doing a good job, so things were not going to change.

***

I was already feeling very insecure, when one morning I woke up and knew something was very wrong. I couldn't understand what was happening.

The whole family were talking about something very serious but were not including me. I was imagining all sorts of things, but mainly, *Are they taking me back to the orphanage?* Kevin, Anthony and Carole did not go to school that day, but I did. I didn't dare question why I was singled out. They had made their decision and that was how it was. Yet again I felt detached from this family.

I was taken to school by a friend of the family who had two younger children, who were not old enough to go to school. He was Catholic. They seemed the only people my mother felt happy to associate with, which was so wrong. Uncle Robert, which is what I was allowed to call him, always seemed a very kind man. He often rode a bicycle across the park to go to church, and I am sure that was how my mother first met him. He allowed me to sit on his handlebars as he took me to school that morning. It was great fun.

My parents were so preoccupied with whatever was going on at home that I don't think they actually noticed me riding off to school on the handlebars, and for a short time it helped me forget my worries.

Dad was standing at the school gate waiting to pick me up that afternoon. I was worried about what he was about to tell me, hoping desperately he was still going to be my father. It was a lovely surprise to see him and I felt very proud to have a parent at the school gate; I was always worried when my mother picked me up in case she said something embarrassing. Dad was much quieter, and didn't get into any conversations with other parents. He just kept himself to himself, which made me feel more relaxed. He smiled as I ran down what seemed a long drive and gave me a hug.

'I couldn't go to work today. I will tell you the reason when we get home but I thought it would be nice to pick you up from school,' he said, which was fine by me! He even bought me some sweets on the way home, which was such a lovely treat.

For now I was enjoying some quality time walking through the park with my dad, being allowed to hold his hand all by myself without Carole doing her best to push her hand through the space to separate our hands. I didn't get told off once, all the way home. I did ask him if I would have to go back to the orphanage. He just laughed and told me not to be so silly. He said, 'We have adopted you and you will be staying with us forever.' That was such a great feeling and I replied, 'Forever and ever?' and he gave me a hug and said, 'Yes, forever and ever'. For a short time I felt so happy and secure.

Dad's whole attitude appeared to change as soon as we got home. Maybe he just did not know how to act under the circumstances. He always tried to please everyone, which is obviously an impossible task, and often his loyalties were torn between his wife and his adopted daughter. In this difficult situation I didn't stand a chance.

As an adopted child your emotions are often intensified and you have to cling to the happier memories, they help you cope with the more difficult things you may have to face. On this occasion I just kept remembering the lovely embrace Dad gave me when I was first introduced to him as my new father, which gave me some comfort.

As we walked through the front door I knew something was terribly wrong as my mother was sitting in a chair crying. But I was not allowed to put my arms around her to give her some comfort, instead I was told to go to my bedroom. I remember Dad putting his finger over my lips to make sure I did not ask any questions. Yet again I was made to feel as if I was not allowed to be involved.

Carole had had the whole day with Mum, so she knew exactly what was happening and the reason why our mother was so upset. As I went to leave the room I saw Carole give her a cuddle and reassure her, saying, 'Don't cry, Gran will soon be better.'

So I found out what was going on by listening to Carole comforting our mother, while I was just told to go to my bedroom as if I had been a naughty girl. As I was going up the stairs I started to cry, and I am not sure if it was because I had been made to feel so left out or if I was upset that our grandmother was so ill. Nobody seemed to understand how I was feeling. It just appeared as if I was a spoilt little girl, crying for attention because she couldn't get her own way.

Dad came upstairs and did at last explain that they had received a telegram from Ireland. 'It tells us that your grandmother has had a stroke and is extremely ill in hospital, so your mother and Carole will be flying to Ireland in the morning.'

***

It had been arranged for Kevin and Anthony to stay with our next-door neighbours, Mr and Mrs Brewin. They did not have any children of their own and enjoyed looking after them. I asked, 'Can't I go to Ireland too, as I will be a really good girl?'

Dad upset me by his reply. He said, 'Carole has to go with her mother, as she will miss her too much, and the boys will be no trouble staying with the neighbours while I'm at work. Anyway, you have only seen your grandmother once and I am sure she will not even know who you are.'

He was usually kinder to me than that, but since Mum was naturally preoccupied with how ill her own mother was, perhaps he felt he had to take over her role and keep me under control. I was told to pack a few things in my small suitcase; the one I had when I left the orphanage over a year ago. I felt like I was going to be sent back to the orphanage. Maybe Dad had lied when he said I would be staying with the family forever. I really thought they had regretted adopting me.

I expect my imagination was getting the better of me. I had just started to feel as if I actually did belong to this family and then suddenly it was all going to be taken away from me. All my memories just came flooding back. I wished I could ask Sister Theresa to help me do my packing, like she did the day I left the orphanage. I was now with a family who did not seem to want me to be there anymore. If they hadn't had me, their lives would have been so much easier. That is how I was made to feel.

The one thing I needed most was the special handkerchief that Sister Theresa had given me, that I had so carelessly lost in the playground on my first day at school. I needed to have something to give me comfort and to wipe away my tears, which by now were running down my face. I had no idea where I was going or how long I would be away, or if I was ever coming back. I was just waiting to be told, sitting on the edge of my bed sobbing my heart out.

Eventually I heard Dad shouting from the bottom of the stairs, 'Phyllis, your tea is ready,' as if it were just an ordinary evening.

I was not in the least bit hungry, but I quickly wiped away my tears, as I knew I would be told off for being selfish and making a fuss.

It was still noticeable that I had been crying as my eyes were red. Dad said, 'You must be strong for your mother as she is already upset, and the last thing she needs is you crying in your soup.' His words seemed so cruel as all I wanted to do was to give Mum a hug to make her pain go away; and it may also have helped my own pain go away.

Kevin and Anthony had already left the house and were having their tea with Mr and Mrs Brewin. Carole actually seemed delighted, as they were flying to Ireland the next day. It was as if they were going on their holidays. Carole was jumping for joy and shouting, 'I have never been in an aeroplane before, we are going to fly high up into the sky.' Apart from when she started school, I had never seen her so excited about anything. I felt she was trying to make me jealous, and she seemed to have forgotten the reason why she was going to Ireland in the first place.

It was as if it was a big adventure instead of going to visit her sick grandmother. Even at such a young age I felt it was being disrespectful to our grandmother, but she never seemed to get told off about anything.

There seemed to be a lot of whispering going on in the house and I was not included. Suddenly I felt really angry and could stand it no longer. If I was going to be sent back to the orphanage I needed to know, so I screamed, 'What is happening to me and where will I be going?' To my amazement I was not reprimanded for screaming out with such anger in my voice.

When I got very upset, my mother seemed to change her attitude towards me and would often take me into another room for a chat, and this is what she did now. She told me that I would be staying with my Auntie Mary, whom I hardly knew.

On one occasion I actually overheard Mum saying to my father, 'I'd better tell her she is special; if not it might cause all sorts of trouble.'

I would be taken into a separate room and she would sit me on her knee, which was a rarity in itself. I would always be extremely embarrassed by the whole thing. Even at such a young age I did not feel my mother was being genuine.

She would always say the same thing. 'We chose you from all the other children at the orphanage because you are special,' but I just wanted to be their daughter, not special. I always felt that was something my mother was advised to say by the nuns when I was first adopted if I became upset. Maybe they thought, if a child feels insecure, by telling them that they are special everything should be just fine.

After having our 'special chats' my mum would always seem to have a self-satisfied and irritating look on her face, as if she had done a great job of making me feel part of the family. If anything, it made me feel even more detached from them all.

Maybe it made her feel less guilty about the way she treated me when she gave me her talks. I don't think she actually believed she was doing anything wrong. She gave the impression that she honestly thought she was the perfect adoptive mother. But at that time all I needed was to feel the same as the rest of the family.

Auntie Mary was my mother's sister in-law; she was married to Uncle Peter, my mother's older brother. They lived on the other side of Birmingham and had four children of their own.

Their house was next door to a primary school, as Uncle Peter was the school caretaker and Auntie Mary was the school cleaner. Kevin was their eldest son and was about 15. He was not in the least bit friendly. He always had his head in a book and just did not seem to want any distractions. Alan was the next cousin. He was

13 and much more into climbing trees and getting into mischief. Kate was the only girl, and just two months younger than Anthony, my brother, so she must have been 11, and by then at secondary school with friends of her own age and not having too much time for her adopted five-year-old cousin.

Then there was Robert, who was a year younger than me. I can only describe him as a male version of Carole, as he spent most of his time trying to get me into trouble, and the rest of the time wishing I wasn't there in the first place. Fortunately this changed in later years and we became quite close.

I remember my mother saying that Auntie Mary had Robert 'in the change'. Obviously at such a young age I had no idea what she actually meant by the change, but I assumed it was something that prevented someone from having any more children of their own. Mum said, 'I suppose it was better to adopt a child than have had one in the change like Auntie Mary did. That would just have been terrible.' I am sure my auntie did not think that; she seemed more than happy to have Robert around.

Even now, when I recall those long six weeks that I stayed there, I remember the pain of loneliness deep in my stomach and the awful feeling of rejection. I was taken early in the morning to my aunt's house by Dad, and I wasn't even allowed to give my mum a farewell hug. Dad told me, 'You said your goodbyes yesterday so let's not make a big fuss today. We need to hurry up as I have got to get back to take your mum and Carole to the airport.' I picked up my suitcase and off we went to my auntie's house. I was a very sad little girl that morning and could tell nobody.

Dad gave me a peck on the cheek and off he went, shouting as he was walking down the path, 'Be a good girl for your Auntie Mary while Mummy and Carole are away in Ireland.' That was the last thing I wanted to hear. My aunt was standing on the doorstep, stern-faced, with Robert by her side. It reminded me of when I first met my mother with her cross face and Carole by her side. I immediately felt once more like an outsider.

I really can't remember too much about my time there. I sometimes think I erased it all from my memory as it was an experience I wanted to forget. I was trying to come to terms with the fact that I had recently been adopted and now I had to stay with an aunt and uncle and their four children, who certainly did not want me there. I am sure that would be too much for any five year old.

I do remember that Dad visited every Saturday afternoon for a couple of hours, and I was constantly being reminded of this, always in a negative way. If I so much as disagreed with anything that was said, my aunt would tell me that I had been disobedient and that my father would be informed of my bad behaviour when he next visited. I would inevitably be punished in some way, usually by being sent to bed. I was made to feel as if I was a naughty child because I had come from an orphanage and was bound to have some behaviour problems.

Meal times were something I came to dread and so I didn't mind being sent to bed. I always had my meals on my own, as if to emphasise the fact that I was not part of their family.

As a small child I hated fried eggs, especially the yolk, but at my aunt's home egg and chips seemed to be on the menu practically every night. I was made to sit at the table until my plate was clean, which often took the whole evening. My aunt would tell me that I should be grateful for the food that is put in front of me and I should think of all the starving children in the world. I would have been more than happy to have shared my fried egg and chips with them. She made me feel like the little girl from the orphanage who was lucky to be given any food at all and did not deserve to be treated any better.

My aunt would say, 'You're not at the orphanage now, so stop feeling so sorry for yourself. I know you have a mind of your own just like your mother.' I never asked if she meant my birth mother or my adoptive mother. I didn't dare. It could have been either of them, as they both had minds of their own, but I'm inclined to think that my adoptive mother would have spoken to my aunt and told her that my birth mother had a strong character, and that is why she was so strict and treated me the way she did, just in case I too got out of control.

I often cried myself to sleep, wishing I was back at the orphanage with Brendan and Sister Theresa to look after me. I did, however, look forward to Saturday afternoons when my dad visited. I suppose I somehow hoped his visits would give me some comfort and reassurance. Auntie Mary would always tell him that I had been a good little girl and I was no trouble. This made me feel so puzzled, Why is she only nice to me on Saturday afternoons? It was so false, but I never told him how I was feeling as he always seemed preoccupied. I would just give him a little smile to make him think that everything was fine.

When Dad did visit I don't recall him speaking about my adoptive mother. It was as if he didn't want to talk about her, so inevitably I would mention her. One visit I asked, 'Is Mummy missing me?'

He paused for a while and then went on to say in an almost dismissive way, 'Well, she has other things on her mind right now, as her own mother is dying.' His words seemed insensitive and cruel, but it got worse.

'Well, at least she has Carole for company, so no, I don't expect she is missing you at the moment.' It was as if he had taken on the role of the dominant parent while she was away but I also realise it was probably an anxious time for him, too. Maybe he just hadn't given too much thought to his adopted daughter's insecurities.

A few weeks went by and my grandmother died. I remember Uncle Peter being very upset as he had been unable to stay in Ireland because of work commitments, but he did manage to get a flight back the following day – in Ireland, funerals are usually the next day.

Robert, who was four, seemed older in the way he acted. Maybe he was just annoyed that I was still around; he really hated me staying at his house. He said, 'My grandmother has died and my daddy will be going to her funeral.'

'My mummy is in Ireland and she will be going to our grandmother's funeral, too,' I replied.

Then he shouted at me angrily, 'Don't be silly, that's not your grandmother. You are adopted so how can you call her your grandmother?'

He was only a small child himself and I suppose it was just the sort of thing children say when they are upset or want to be mean to each other. But at the time it really affected me, and I remember crying about what he had said and my aunt asking me in her usual abrupt manner what I was crying about. I didn't tell her. I knew it would be pointless.

On the last day at my aunt's house I overheard her talking to Mrs Evans, a woman I didn't know who had called at the house. My aunt hadn't realised that I was reaching to get my coat, thinking it would be better if I went into the garden to get out of the way. In the hall-way there stood a circular stand so laden with coats that it seemed to defy gravity and I was well concealed.

She stood there with her arms folded under her large bosom. She had a habit of taking hankies from her multi-coloured print overall and dabbing her face, usually saying something along the lines of 'it's my age, you know'. She was not letting Mrs Evans get a word in edgeways, and in the middle of the non-stop flow of words I suddenly heard her say, 'I mean, if I would have wanted to adopt a child I could have gone to the orphanage myself. I already have four children of my own. Doesn't her mother think I have enough to be doing?'

I froze on the spot. This confirmed what I already knew to be true. I wanted to run away, maybe even go back to the orphanage, as I felt scared, unloved and certainly unwanted. I was convinced that my adoptive parents regretted ever going to the orphanage in the first place, let alone adopting me.

The next day I was taken back to my adoptive family. It felt like I was going to a new place and I had to start all over again. My mother was grieving for her own mother but at the time I was just too young to understand. When she seemed sad I would feel rejected and just go to my bedroom and cry myself to sleep.

I never did tell anyone how upset I felt at my aunt's house. They didn't ask me any questions and I had learnt very quickly to keep things to myself. I knew then that I had to grow up fast, and being too sensitive about things wasn't going to help me. I decided to try my best to be a good girl so I wouldn't get into trouble and just maybe they would learn to love me as their own daughter.

Chapter 3

Growing Up

Back with my family, I tried to put the fact that I had been adopted to the back of my mind. I was desperate just to feel that I belonged, and that they were happy to have me as their daughter and sister. I just wanted to be a normal little girl and to be treated the same as the other children. Not special in any way.

But my adoptive mother always made me feel that she didn't want me to be part of the family. She certainly did not consider how an adopted child might be affected by the insensitive comments she so often made.

One of her most tactless habits was to talk constantly about the times when she was expecting her children.

She would go into great detail about her pregnancies: how long she was in labour, what the midwife was like and how much the babies weighed. Even what the weather was like on the day they were born. She would mention how long she had breast-fed them and the fact that her milk was too watery and it did not have enough nutrients. I mean, does a six-year-old girl really need to have such detail? I obviously felt excluded from these conversations and jealous that I would never be given such information about my birth or first days and months.

When children are given this kind of knowledge by their birth parents they just absorb it, and may even become bored by it, but as an adopted child it can be quite painful to be denied it. You desperately want to be told about every minute detail so you can form your own identity and feel more secure as a young child growing up. Thankfully, with the Freedom of Information Act now in place, adopted children are given these details about themselves.

My adoptive mother would often talk about another couple who had also wanted to give me a home. They had no children of their own and lived in Coventry. On one occasion, when she was annoyed by something that I had done, she shouted at me and said, 'Maybe things would have been better if you had been adopted by the other couple. Then they would have spoilt you, which is what you expect from me.'

But I never wanted to be spoilt. I just wanted to be loved and not to feel rejected by them. I felt like shouting back, Yes, maybe they would have spoilt me like you spoil Carole, but I would have only been in more trouble so I always kept that thought to myself.

She went on to tell me (maybe she was feeling slightly guilty by her first comment) that the nuns always felt I would be better placed within a family with brothers and sisters, since I was a chatterbox and obviously needed company.

However, having a sister like Carole, who seemed to spend most of her time trying to get me into trouble and the rest of her time just not wanting me to be there anyway, was not the kind of company I actually needed. I often felt upset and lonely. I daydreamed about 'the lady from Coventry', thinking that it might actually be my birth mother.

The one thing I did know from an early age was that I had been born in Coventry. This was on my small birth certificate, the only document I was ever allowed to see about myself.

This record didn't tell me much. It had been re-registered in 1960, following my adoption, with my surname registered as theirs. Phyllis Price – it felt like the previous four years of my life had never existed. I only had my own memories of what my life was like pre-adoption.

I had been told that my birth father had died from TB when I was six months old, and my birth mother six months later from the same illness. However, I guessed she probably still lived in Coventry. In my heart I knew she was alive.

One evening, when she seemed to be in a good mood, I felt the time was right to ask why I had been placed for adoption. I was then about ten and, I suppose, becoming more curious about why my birth mother had given me up.

I took a deep breath and went on to ask whether the main reason I had been adopted was because my mother had a baby before she was married. This was something I had in mind since, as I went to a Catholic school, the main part of our sex education was that you must get married before you have a child. We were told it was a mortal sin to conceive out of wedlock.

She was very firm in her reply. 'Of course your mother was married. She was not that type of woman,' whatever that was supposed to mean.

I went on to ask whether it was unusual for both my mother and father to have died so young and within six months of each other. By now her patience was running out. She shouted, 'What is it with all the questions? I've told you before that your mother and father are dead, so let that be an end to it!'

I left the room and listened at the door, and sure enough she started talking about me. She said, 'One day that child will get really hurt. I think we have done the right thing by saying her parents have both died as the last thing we want is for her to turn out like her own mother.'

I had such mixed emotions, it was hard for me to take it all in. But the one thing I do remember thinking to myself was, I can't be hurt any more than how my adoptive mother has already hurt me. It made me even more determined to discover the truth one day. I realised it was not the right time to ask any more questions of my adoptive parents. Maybe there would never be a right time.

One Sunday morning I felt unwell and didn't go to Mass. Later on in the afternoon I was feeling much better, full of beans and playing with my skipping rope. I was promptly marched off to evening Mass for telling such terrible fibs, even though it actually wasn't a lie. I hadn't felt well in the morning. But she wasn't in any mood to listen to my explanation.

I felt so angry. How can anyone be so hypocritical? She was annoyed with me for telling lies, yet she told me so many about my adoption. I felt like shouting, You're always telling lies. I know my mother is really alive and I know she never married my father.

Not that it made the slightest difference to me whether I was conceived in or out of wedlock. It was just the fact that it was all right for her to lie, but if she suspected me of doing the same I was humiliated and marched off to the confession box. It just didn't seem fair.

When we went to church on Sundays, during the Mass you would pray for the souls of people who had gone before us. I would always say a little prayer for my mother, hoping that one day I would be able to meet her. This helped me cope.

Sometimes we visited Coventry Cathedral on Sunday afternoons, as in those days all the shops were closed and Sundays were very quiet. It made me feel sad that I was visiting my birthplace, but that was all I knew. It did, however, make me feel closer to my birth mother.

I remember asking if I could light a candle for the 'sick people', as I wanted to try to make them feel better. Dad smiled and gave me some coins to put in the collection box. By this time I was starting to think how much I wanted to be a nurse when I grew up, which was something Dad encouraged.

I lit the candle and prayed for my birth mother, asking God to take care of her. It was as if I had made some kind of connection with her. Even at such a young age, I found it difficult to understand, but I always feared that she was in danger and needed my prayers.

It was the only thing at the time that I could do for her. I feared that she might be coming to some harm and that she was not happy, but I was helpless and had nobody to talk to about my feelings. The only thing at that time was to pray that her guardian angel would take care of her and keep her from harm. Saying a prayer gave me some comfort, as at least I had told God. I am sure my prayers were answered as she was protected from harm on so many occasions. She was often in very dangerous situations – drunk and lying in gutters, almost choking on her own vomit – but somehow she survived against all the odds.

***

When things are not going too well with their new families, some adoptive children imagine their birth mother to be perfect. In my heart I always knew this wasn't the case for me, and I am sure these feelings somehow sowed a seed in me of wanting to help people. This decision, which I never wavered from (and is the job I still do today), certainly helped me to deal with what I had to face when I did eventually meet my birth mother. It also helped shape the person I became.

Perhaps my adoptive mother was trying to protect me from finding out about my birth mother, hoping that I would just accept the fact that she had died, but adopted children deserve to be told the truth about themselves. It is a fundamental human right to be given information about your origins, whether good or bad. Children are much more resilient than we give them credit for, and it is far better to be told the truth so that eventually they can come to terms with it.

It is worse being told nothing. You feel detached from your adoptive parents as in any close relationship trust plays a major part. It somehow makes you feel incomplete as a person.

***

When I was 11 and leaving primary school I was happy that I would no longer be with Pauline, the girl who had often bullied me about being adopted. Thankfully she was going to a different secondary school. I was determined to put her threats behind me. She wouldn't be able to hurt me anymore, and I decided that I wasn't going to tell another soul.

It was now July 1967 and I was looking forward to the summer holidays, which were to include some of the happiest childhood memories I can remember. We were going to Cornwall, and staying in a caravan close to the sea.

I was so looking forward to it, as previously we had always gone to Ireland on holiday, usually just visiting relatives, so this was going to be something totally different. Dad had just passed his driving test and had managed to save enough money to buy a car. Kevin, now aged 20, had also thrown away his L plates the previous year and had a car, so it was all very exciting.

Kevin had a girlfriend called Sheila who was allowed to come on holiday with us. My adoptive mother always encouraged Kevin to have girlfriends. He was a boy, and her natural child at that, so he wouldn't bring shame on the family. Or so she thought.

Mum seemed to feel sorry for Sheila and would always try to make a fuss of her. She made a point of telling me how most of Sheila's childhood had been spent in a children's home, although sometimes she did stay with foster parents and her older brother. Her birth mother had left when she was five, and that was something, my mum said, she had never really recovered from.

While trying to impress Kevin's girlfriend, Mum intermittently whispered to me how fortunate I was to have been adopted by them. 'Otherwise you would have been in the children's home until you were 17, just like Sheila.' She was right of course, and I am grateful for that – although it was something that she never allowed me to forget.

But for now I was on holiday and having a good time. I spent many hours building sandcastles with the bucket and spade that had been left in the caravan by the previous occupants. I was lost in my imaginary world and enjoying every minute of it. I was so happy; I felt like any other little girl on the beach spending time with her family on holiday. To the outside world that was exactly what it looked like, but deep down I knew we were far from being an ordinary family. I tried hard not to dwell on something that was not going to change.

One evening I was feeling unwell and wanting to go back to the caravan so I could have a sleep. Mum shouted, 'No. Kevin and Sheila are there and need some privacy.' We walked for what seemed like ages and I was not allowed to go back into the caravan until it was dark. I was just told to stop moaning as 'you don't come on holiday to sit in the caravan all night'.

Can you believe that when we actually got back into the caravan my mother whispered, 'Isn't it nice to see Kevin giving Sheila a cuddle on the sofa, as I'm sure she didn't have much love at the children's home?' I so felt like shouting, I really would like to have a cuddle from my mum as I don't feel well.

I just went to bed and kept my thoughts to myself because the last thing I wanted was one of her 'special chats'. The one thing I certainly did not feel that night was 'special'. I don't think she actually believed she was doing anything wrong. She gave the impression that she honestly thought she was the perfect adoptive mother. But at that time all I needed was a cuddle.

The holiday came to an end and I started secondary school and made some new friends. I knew I would not be telling them about my adoption. I had learnt my lesson from my previous experiences, and did not want to spend the rest of my time at school in fear of anyone finding out. I had to keep that secret to myself.

One Saturday afternoon, early in September 1967, it was still quite warm so I was playing in the garden. I would play for hours, totally lost in my imaginary world – my favourite game involved my dolls and my clapped-out bicycle. I called it the Dolls' and Teds' Bus Stop Game. We had a big garden and I would leave little markings as the stops on the route, with the dolls and teddies in the basket on the back of the bike. I had an old handbag over my shoulder with tickets from a post office game I had from Father Christmas years before. I would pick up and drop off my dolls and teddies at different bus stops. I don't expect children would be too impressed with my game today, but for me as a child then it was great fun. At least it kept me out of trouble.

I was totally absorbed in my made-up game when I suddenly heard Dad shouting at the top of his voice. I noticed Kevin and Sheila were there, but it was rare for him to be shouting if we had a visitor. I put my bicycle down on the lawn and ran inside to see what all the commotion was about. Mum immediately shouted at me, 'This has nothing to do with you. Go back into the garden.'

I had painful pangs of jealousy, knowing Carole was allowed to stay in the house and I'd been ordered out. I went back in the garden and carried on playing my favourite game, but not really concentrating on it as I was hurting so much. I knew it must be something serious as there was a lot of shouting, and usually if we had a visitor Mum would put on a show and act as if everything was just fine.

By now it was getting late and I was starting to feel cold, shivering as I hadn't got a cardigan on. I was unsure what to do, as I knew I would be shouted at if I attempted to go back into the house. Eventually Anthony came out into the garden and almost seemed excited about the rumpus. 'You'll never guess what's happened,' and, not giving me even a second to guess, continued, 'Sheila is pregnant and Mum and Dad are going crazy.' I said, 'But it'll be nice to have a baby in the family.' And Anthony replied, 'Yes, but they're not married, and Mum is worried about what the neighbours will think.' I suddenly didn't feel quite so cold.

***

Within a month the wedding had been arranged. I said to Mum, 'What's all the rush about? Why can't they wait until the baby is born?' Yet again I was shouted at for speaking my mind, which so often got me into all sorts of trouble.

'Absolutely not, 'she said, 'it's only really bad girls who have a baby before they are married and that sort of girl should be ashamed of themselves.' Of course she immediately blamed Sheila, and contradicted everything that she had said while we were on holiday in July. She talked quite openly about how the baby was conceived and started to get annoyed with the fact that they had been given too much time by themselves when we were on holiday. I couldn't help thinking about the time when I felt so ill and wasn't allowed to go back to the caravan as Kevin and Sheila needed time by themselves. I was certainly not going to remind her of that!

I knew my birth mother was single when I was conceived. I don't know why I was so sure. Maybe it was the fact that it was always emphasised that she was married that made me so convinced that she wasn't. When my adoptive mother was telling lies she would often repeat her statements several times as if to emphasise the fact that she was telling the 'truth'. She would look across at my adoptive father and give him one of her stern looks as if to dare him to disagree, as 'this is what Phyllis must believe'.

Now, she said that Sheila tricked Kevin into getting her pregnant. She must have led him on, and then he just couldn't control himself. It was as if Kevin had played no part in what had happened. The fact that Kevin was just 20 and Sheila was only 17 was not the issue. The only thing that she seemed concerned about was 'what will the neighbours think?'

The wedding went ahead in October 1967 and Sheila was due to give birth in April 1968.

Two months before the baby arrived Kevin and Sheila had a small collision with another car. Thankfully, nobody was hurt, but Mum said it was a Godsend. She was able to seize the opportunity to tell yet more lies. Mum decided to tell everyone that the collision had caused the baby to arrive two months early, and then hopefully nobody would realise that Sheila had been pregnant before they got married.

The problem with telling lies is you need to have a good memory and some knowledge about what you are actually lying about. Mum had neither of these. She often got the facts all wrong and would go into great detail about everything, trying to make herself be believed. She told the next door neighbour how the baby was born with no nails, and had no eyebrows or eyelashes. Our neighbour at the time did have a confused look on her face, and it was only years later when I was at college doing my pre-nursing course that I realised why. I had done a project on childcare and learnt all about how a baby develops in the womb. In the last two months the foetus just needs to grow, and if it does arrive early it would be underweight but fully developed. So Mum's lies, intended to cover up something that she felt would bring shame on the family, only exposed her further.

She was a compulsive liar. Mum would lie about anything just to ensure we appeared as a 'respectable' family. What I think she failed to realise was that the neighbours were just ordinary people going about their own lives and not at all interested in what our family were actually doing. I often thought to myself, Why can't she just enjoy the birth of her first grandchild? But Mum never seemed to see things for how they were, and she would always have to complicate everything.

Chapter 4

My Teenage Years

Although I was only a child I often felt much wiser than my adoptive mother. This would land me in all sorts of trouble, often questioning what she had said, which was something the rest of the family never did – usually to keep the peace! It is difficult to have a conversation with someone who always thinks they are right in whatever they say.

I was now allowed to go home by myself. Mrs Brewin, our next door neighbour, had no children of her own and seemed to enjoy having a chat with me when I came home from school. I think she had a soft spot for me and may have felt a little upset about how I was sometimes treated.

She was an elderly lady now, and just seemed to want someone to talk to. She was a little confused, but she never forgot the time I would be getting home from school. Weather permitting, she would be in her front garden doing some weeding, hoping for a little chat. She often gave me sweets, which I would quickly hide in my pocket. It always seemed to anger Mum if anyone ever gave me too much attention. More often than not Mrs Brewin would ask me if I'd had a nice day at school and had I learnt anything interesting. It was so nice to have someone who was actually curious about what I was doing.

Even then I loved talking to older people. Their stories of the war years fascinated me. Our chats seemed to brighten up her day, and I did feel really sorry for her as she seemed so lonely. Most of her day was spent indoors looking after her frail husband, who had suffered from a stroke that affected his speech and needed full-time nursing care.

I often heard her say, 'My Charlie's not going into an old people's home,' which is what they called care homes in those days. The district nurses visited twice a day and I thought to myself how I would love to do their job when I was older, nursing sick people in their own homes and maybe preventing them from having to go into hospital.

Whenever I was speaking to Mrs Brewin my mum

would try and get my attention by calling me from the window. Her stern expression gave me butterflies in my stomach.

Sometimes I would defy her and spend even more time talking, knowing full well that I would be in greater trouble when I did eventually go inside. Making an old lady's day a little brighter seemed to be more important to me at the time. Inevitably when I did go back into the house my adoptive mother would be furious and start shouting, 'Why are you telling her all our family secrets? She only talks to you because she knows you will tell her all our business. She doesn't talk to Carole as she knows she is more sensible and loyal to the family and wouldn't give our secrets away.'

She was so cruel at times; I remember feeling confused and sad. What was so bad about being friendly and kind to a lonely old lady who didn't even ask any questions about the 'family secrets', whatever they may have been on that particular day? What annoyed me the most was that Carole just could not be bothered with older people, and would totally ignore Mrs Brewin whenever she said 'hello', which was so unfriendly. I felt I needed to overcompensate for her rudeness.

***

I was growing up and I suppose I had quite a strong personality. Sometimes I just needed to express myself as an individual. I was always being compared with Carole, and never favourably. No matter what I did, it was wrong.

I recall one evening being late home from school. On the way home an old lady had been getting off the bus when she slipped and hurt her ankle. The poor thing had two heavy bags of shopping, and her apples started rolling down the bus. She was really struggling and nobody seemed bothered to try to help her. The other children just laughed and called her names. I felt so angry; how could they be so cruel to such a helpless old lady? I quickly picked up some of the escaping apples and jumped off the bus.

It wasn't my stop, but I didn't care. I was worried about how she was going to manage on her own. She seemed upset and in a lot of pain, and for a moment I forgot that I would be in trouble for being late home from school. Unsurprisingly, Carole had stayed on the bus, and was shouting at me to get back on. I shouted back to her, 'Tell Mum I am helping the lady with her heavy bags, as she has hurt herself.'

I carried the lady's bags as we walked slowly to her house. Although my arms were aching it was worth it to see the smile on her face as we reached her front door. She was so grateful for my help and didn't appear to be in as much pain from her ankle. I remember her saying, 'What a lovely girl you are for helping me. Your mother must be so proud of you'.

I just smiled politely and kept my thoughts to myself, knowing full well that my mother was anything but proud of me. I cried on the way home, partly because I was scared about being told off for being late home from school. I knew Carole would have conveniently forgotten to mention what had happened. But I also felt upset because of what the old lady had said about my mother being proud of me.

Sure enough, I was told off and sent to bed early that night. I was not even given the chance to explain what I had been doing. I am not sure to this day what Carole's explanation was of why I was so late home from school that evening, but she always made sure that she was seen in the best light. My mother shouted at me, 'Why can't you be a good girl like your sister and mind your own business? Then you would manage to get home on time like her.'

There were so many occasions when I was told off for something that I hadn't even done. I was always seen as the naughty one. I'm sure sometimes I was, but Carole was certainly no angel. I can't recall her ever being told off about anything in the whole of our childhood. She was the one who was made to feel 'special', not me.

I enjoyed secondary school, even though I was often getting told off by the nuns for talking too much in class. The nuns were very strict. Their long cream habits, with their veils cut squarely around their faces, reminded me of my time spent at the orphanage. But there was nobody there as kind as my beloved Sister Theresa.

Carole was the complete opposite to me in her personality as well as the way she looked. She was very quiet and mainly kept herself to herself. From what I can remember she only seemed to have one main friend, who was the smallest in her class and seemed quite sweet – I somehow felt sorry for her. I am unsure what Carole actually told her about me; but she did not want to be a friend of mine.

At break times they would sit on their usual bench, not mixing with other classmates, so they were often seen as being quite aloof.

Carole was known as a 'goody-goody'. I dread to think what I was known as, but I was certainly more talkative than Carole and, I suppose against all the odds, I found it much easier to make friends. Carole always gave me the feeling that she was ashamed to have me as her sister and would distance herself from me when we were at school − or at any other time, come to think of it. We were not close, and I wasn't that pleased about having her as my sister, either.

I remember one afternoon we were having our photographs taken at school and the nuns had arranged for these to be taken with our siblings, which did not usually happen in secondary schools.

As it was Christmas time they thought it would be a special treat for our parents, although, as my adoptive mother had said, it was just an unnecessary expense at this already expensive time. The older girls at the school had to collect any younger sisters. I was so embarrassed when Carole walked into the classroom to collect me. Suddenly the whole class just gasped and once again one of the girls shouted out, 'That can't be your sister! They must have mixed up the babies in the hospital!'

This caused great laughter and the nun who was teaching that particular class very quickly clapped her hands together to tell the class to be quiet. When I went home from school that day I was upset at the comments that had been made and blurted out, 'I don't look like anyone and I don't feel part of this family.' If ever I got too upset like that, and as long as Carole was not involved, my adoptive mother would try in her own clumsy way to make things better.

A friend of hers from the church called at the house in the evening. I could hear them both whispering, and I suspected it was about me. Sure enough, my suspicions were confirmed when I was called to the front door. The woman gave me a sympathetic smile as if she knew my whole life story. Knowing what my adoptive mother was like, I'm sure she actually did. I remember her suddenly talking really loud as if she was trying to reinforce what she was saying. It was like something from a script, and so well-rehearsed.

Her friend looked at me and said, 'Phyllis, you look so like your mum. You have her nose.' I felt so embarrassed, but she went on relentlessly, adding, '... and you certainly have her eyes and her chin.' By the time she was finished I was the complete double of my mother, which I knew was not the case. It was so obvious that my adoptive mother had told her everything about my adoption and how I was upset about not resembling any of the family, even though it was meant to be the best-kept family secret. It just made me feel worse as I knew I looked nothing like them.

I felt so patronised by her but had to pretend that I was reassured by her comments. Later on my adoptive mother appeared smug and reminded me of what the woman had said, 'See you do look like me. Even the lady from the church had noticed, so it must be true.'

This just made me feel more frustrated. Did she really believe I was so gullible as to be reassured by what a complete stranger had said? On the positive side, as I got older I was secretly quite glad that I didn't actually resemble any of my adoptive family. My mother always dealt with anything to do with my adoption by telling lies and even got other people to lie for her if she thought it would help convince me about something. But the irony of it all was I never was convinced; she just thought I was.

There was another instance that stands out. It was one sunny afternoon when we were playing rounders in the playground and wearing our summer T-shirts. One of the known bullies was looking at us both and shouted, 'I think Phyllis has got her sister's share in the bosom area as Carole is as flat as a pancake.' This caused a group of the girls to giggle but for myself and Carole it caused great embarrassment.

My body was changing. Puberty was well and truly kicking in, and the one thing I did not want to happen, did. My body changed sooner than Carole's, even though I was 18 months younger. My breasts were developing sooner than Carole's, but for weeks it just wasn't mentioned.

I was starting to feel very self-conscious, particularly when doing PE at school, and eventually I plucked up the courage to ask if I could have a bra. Mum sighed and said, 'But I haven't even bought Carole one yet, and I hope you realise they are very expensive to buy.' Not exactly what you expect your mother's reply to be.

Eventually she did buy me a bra but it certainly was not the best experience. I remember actually being told off for wearing a T-shirt. 'It is far too clingy and you will make Carole feel self-conscious,' she screamed. I felt like shouting back, 'She isn't wearing the T-shirt. I am.'

She did not consider that, as the well-developed one, I may be the one feeling a bit embarrassed. I knew that would just land me in even bigger trouble, so I kept the thought to myself. She was annoyed that I had bigger boobs than Carole, which just confirmed what I already knew: she resented having me as her daughter. How else could her bizarre outburst be explained?

Following that comment I usually wore big loose jumpers so that I would not be drawing attention to myself. 'Showing off' was how she described it.

I was often upset by her cruel words, usually over-hearing what she was saying when I listened outside the door. Needless to say I eventually stopped doing this as I never liked what I heard and became almost paranoid about myself, particularly where my body image was concerned. It had long been obvious that Carole was the favourite, but my teenage years were even harder to deal with. I used to think to myself, Why did they adopt me?

Inevitably, I also started my periods a few months before Carole. I had been really dreading them anyway – the first period is when a daughter needs her mother's support, and not to be made to feel like some freak. I remember not wanting to tell Mum as I was so worried about what her reaction might be.

I wondered how to bring up the subject and then thought of a good plan. We had two poodles, so it was always a big thing when they were 'in season'. They were not allowed to be taken for a walk in case a dog came sniffing around.

Having the poodles neutered was against the Catholic religion and for years I always thought this was really silly. We don't take them to church so why do they have to follow the faith? It always seemed so cruel that we were not allowed to take the dogs for a walk, as they were desperate to get out of the house and do what comes naturally. I'm sure it sent them crazy.

Having dogs was how I explained about my periods. It's rather amusing that the poodles being in season was something that was so often mentioned but girls starting their periods was ignored. I picked a moment when my mother seemed to be in a good mood, which I always had to do if I needed to broach a sensitive subject.

The main worry was that I had started my periods before Carole and I knew that would not please her. I just blurted it out. 'Mum I think I'm in season,' which was a funny way of putting it.

She smiled, and I suppose it did break the ice. 'Does that mean I will have to stay in the house the same as the dogs?' I asked. I remember my mother's reply, as she said it in a kind of jokey way, but certainly with a serious side to it, 'Yes, you will need to keep away from the boys now as the last thing we want to happen is for you to get pregnant. You don't want to have to give your baby up for adoption.'

That remark still takes my breath away. I really could not get over how insensitive she was. But my mum just looked worried, as if she was thinking to herself, Well this is when the problems start. For me, the result was that I was scared stiff of ever being left alone with a boy but totally unsure of what might actually happen if I was!

I attended an all girls' convent school, and was never allowed to go out with any of my friends at the week-end, so keeping away from the boys was not that diffi-cult. Even a trip to the cinema for a few hours was out of the question. I really felt hurt that she had no trust in me as her daughter. A few days after I told her about my periods, true to character she seemed put out, saying, 'I can't believe I am going to have the expense of buying you sanitary towels before Carole.'

She went on to attempt (rather comically) to explain about the birds and the bees. She said that, 'Boys might get the wrong idea. If you hold their hand they will think you are ready to have sex with them. Boys cannot control their feelings, so the girl must be strong and stay in control, and not give them the least bit of encouragement. Even a smile can give them the wrong idea.'

I really thought that women had no pleasure when having sex, and was very confused about the whole situation of ever having a boyfriend. I am glad to say that eventually I did realise what my mother had told me was nonsense, and thankfully I found the majority of boys to be far from how she perceived them.

Mum had some strange ideas about sex. Partly because of her faith, and partly because she was convinced that I was going to be as sexually active as my birth mother. Of course, she was unable to say this since she had already told me that my birth mother had died from TB and had supposedly been married to my father. Everything seemed respectable, so how could she mention anything to the contrary?

She was so strict with me as a teenager and I always knew there was something else that she was trying to hide from me. My birth mother was more than just an unmarried mother. I knew asking her any questions was going to be a complete waste of energy so I would have to be patient. But I was determined that one day I would find out the truth.

In the meantime I had to pretend to believe everything I had been told. My mother and father were married and had both died. Sometimes I was tempted to complicate matters and ask where my parents were buried, and demand to be taken to their graves. But, again, this would have been a pointless exercise as I would have been given some silly excuse and would have to pretend to believe it.

When I was 14 years old I had one of my favourite holidays ever, and that was because I went on holiday with my dad all by myself. We were going to Blackpool for a whole week and stayed in a bed and breakfast. Carole and Mum had gone the week before – staying in the same guest house. Mum never liked putting the poodles in kennels so she decided we should take separate holidays, which was fine by me.

It was lovely to spend a whole week just with Dad. The weather wasn't too good, we had a few rainy and windy days, but that didn't dampen our holiday spirits.

After breakfast we would spend a couple of hours on the beach. I was acting younger than my years, I really was like a little girl on holiday with her daddy. I never got told off about anything, he was always happy to be with me and I really did enjoy spending time with him. I was shown so much love.

We had an afternoon at the fun fair and I even persuaded Dad to go on the Big Dipper, though he looked terrified when he got off. We laughed about it all afternoon with the help of the laughing clown – you put the money in the machine and just stand watching the clown laughing till eventually you couldn't stop laughing yourself. We went in the haunted house where there were cobwebs blowing in Dad's face which made him jump out of his skin, then he saw me jump when I saw myself as a little fat figure in the funny mirrors.

We laughed so much on that holiday we had a stitch in our side. On the way home we sat on the wall tucking into fish and chips only for the seagulls to fly down and steal most of my fish.

Dad just laughed and said, 'I suppose you want some of my fish now.' With a giggle I nodded my head. To make up for losing my fish Dad bought me a T-shirt with my name printed on it, and the rest of the holiday we always sat inside to eat our fish and chips. That is a holiday I will never forget. I really was Daddy's little girl! I love you, Dad.

***

Mum tried to put me off being a nurse as she hated anything to do with illness, but Dad encouraged me.

I was in my last year at school and often studying in the bedroom, busy revising for my exams. I knew I had to work hard as I wanted to become a nurse. One evening I was in bed, almost falling asleep over my books, when I heard a crackling noise. At first I thought it was Anthony messing about by actually walking up the stairs with a sparkler in his hand! Then I could smell smoke, to my horror I could see the smoke coming from under the door. I ran out of the bedroom, and as I ran past the flames that were coming from the airing cupboard my long hair set alight. I ran down the stairs in sheer fright, shouting, 'FIRE!' I grabbed a towel from the downstairs toilet, which I wrapped around my head, while Dad phoned the fire service and shouted for everyone to get out.

Standing in the front garden, Mum told my dad to get some valuables out of the house, so poor Dad ran back into the house and came out with the Yellow Pages from the phone table. Mum was not impressed!

The firemen arrived in no time and soon set about putting the fire out. I was shivering as I only had a short nylon nightie on. One of the firemen kindly wrapped his heavy jacket around me and Mum said, 'My other daughter would have thought to put on her coat. But this one, well she doesn't think, she's too busy flirting with you lot.'

I was speechless, but the fireman just gave me a friendly wink and said, 'Don't worry, love, as long as you're OK.'

Things continued to become more difficult as I got older. Relatives and friends would often say in a jokey way, 'You don't look like your sister, you're better looking.' This was the last thing my adoptive mother wanted to hear. It made me feel very uncomfortable and made Carole even more resentful.

My brother Anthony was getting married and his fiancé picked two bridesmaids both with blonde hair – one of them was me. For the first time, at the age of 16, I was picked to do something without Carole being asked first. It was very strange, I had never felt anything but second best before. It was amazing, but mostly I was anxious it would have some repercussions with Carole and my mum. I also wondered why you should have to look a certain way to be accepted. Sadly that's just how things are sometimes.

***

When I was 17 our cousin James from America, who was about ten years older than me, came to stay with us for a few weeks. I remember him being very kind to me but he did not seem to take much notice of Carole. He always seemed to look at me the way a boy does when he finds a girl attractive. He told me he found it difficult to talk to girls as he was shy, but he found it easy to chat to me and he enjoyed my company.

Carole, James and I were all going out to a local disco. It was the first time I had ever been allowed to do anything like that and I remember being very excited. Carole had lipstick on, so I asked if I could wear some too. Not surprisingly I was told, 'You can't, as lipstick takes the colour out of your lips.' I remember thinking, has Carole not got any colour in her lips?

When we arrived at the disco, Carole met a friend from school and James asked me to dance. He was dancing very close to me, which made me feel uncomfortable, and he whispered in my ear in his American accent, 'Do you know you are one very attractive young lady and I so wish you were not my cousin.' Then he thought for a while and said, 'You know you are too pretty to be a Price, but come to think of it you're not a real Price.'

I suppose I should have been flattered that he found me attractive, but I felt confused and upset. It highlighted the fact that once again I did not feel part of this family. I kept my distance from him for the rest of his visit, as the last thing I wanted was for Mum to know about his comments. I was sure she would have been convinced that I had given him some type of encouragement.

I was rarely allowed to wash my hair and as a teenager it was often very greasy. I would be told some silly old wives' tales like, 'You can't wash your hair, as it will wash away all your own natural oils.' I suppose it was a bit like the lipstick.

It was only as I got older that it dawned on me, the last thing my adoptive mother wanted was for me to look more attractive than Carole. I suppose that if I didn't wash my hair or wear lipstick, she hoped that would be the case. Actually, Carole had lovely brown curly hair, and if only she had stopped being aloof and chatted to people I'm sure she'd have been thought attractive.

At the time I can't help thinking about the fairy tale of Cinderella. Not for one minute am I saying Carole is an 'ugly sister', but in this story the mother and her natural daughters were jealous of Cinderella and kept her in rags, simply because they perceived her as being prettier. Daft as it sounds, I really related to this story. I often had to wear hand-me-downs, but Carole would be bought new clothes.

Carole left school and went on a short hand typing course, coming home for her lunch and after work every day. She started going out to the pubs in town with a friend from work. Mum encouraged me to join them, which I did a couple of times, but if I as much as gave a boy a peck on the cheek it would be reported back to Mum, so I thought it was easier to just let Carole go out with her own friends.

When I left school, a friend and I went into a clothes shop up the road to ask about a job, and we got it there and then. I worked there for six weeks before I went to college, and then on Saturdays. Finally I had a little bit of money, and as well as giving my parents some rent I was able to buy myself some new outfits.

It was nice to dress up when I went to college. I realised I needed to concentrate on my pre-nursing course – but my friend Ann was keen to rush down to the canteen at lunchtime to start chatting to the new lads on the plumbing and electrical courses. I was more than happy to accompany her.

It was my first taste of independence and I loved it. I started seeing a boy with curly blond hair called Sam – my first boyfriend! But how would Mum react?

We went on a few dates and he seemed lovely. He was mad on football and was a Villa supporter, so I went to my first football match. I also went to his house to meet his dad and little sister. Sadly his mum had died the year before, so I tried to give him some comfort.

He hadn't been to my house and it was something I was dreading. One night there was a knock on the door and there was Sam standing outside. He thought he would surprise me, which he certainly did. I grabbed my jacket and shouted to Mum as I left, 'Just going for a walk in the park!'

We held hands as couples do and enjoyed a lovely spring evening. As Sam was giving me a rather passionate good night kiss, Mum suddenly appeared at the front gate and shouted, 'Don't forget about the dogs!'

Sam now looked confused but trying to be helpful said, 'Do you want me to walk your dogs?'

'NO!' Mum replied sharply. 'Phyllis knows what I mean.' She grabbed my arm and pulled me into the house.

I was so embarrassed by the whole incident, particularly when Sam asked about taking the poodles out the next time I saw him. The romance ended rather abruptly.

Chapter 5

Nurse Training

I'd always wanted to be a nurse since I was a little girl. It appealed to me to be doing a job that would make a difference to people's lives by helping them through difficult times, for instance recovering from illness. Nursing has enabled me to do that and more.

When I was just 17 I completed a pre-nursing course at college and passed – first class! Feeling very proud of myself, I then applied to become a cadet nurse, and was accepted on a course, subject to a successful medical.

Unfortunately this raised questions like, 'Are there any hereditary illnesses we need to know about?' When I said that I was adopted it stopped the conversation dead. I was so nervous. Firstly, I hadn't spoken about my adoption to anyone since I'd been bullied in primary school. Secondly, I was wondering whether I should mention that I had been told both my natural parents had died of TB. I decided to say nothing, as this version of my parentage never rang true anyway.

My worries disappeared when I received a letter from the School of Nursing at Dudley Road Hospital, which informed me that I had been accepted on to the cadet course. By the summer of 1973 I started working on the wards, gaining practical experience before attending college. Three out of the five days we studied for our GCE O levels.

As cadet nurses we weren't expected to work late shifts, weekends, nights or bank holidays, and for six months we worked Monday to Friday from 9 a.m. till 4 p.m., usually being allowed to finish at 3.30 p.m. on Friday afternoons. This, however, depended on the ward sister you got.

It was an enjoyable time in my life and being adopted was something I rarely even thought about. I was young, doing a job that I loved and had made a lot of new friends. They were from various religions with different beliefs, and all pleasant and friendly with each other. I had the opportunity of meeting lots of other people my own age who were not Catholic. It was a great feeling.

***

There were two incidents during this period that I have only just realised were significant.

When I started working at the hospital I travelled on the number 11 bus, which went around the outer circle of Birmingham. I usually caught the bus at about eight in the morning, giving me plenty of time to be on the wards by nine.

I will always remember my first ward, which was 'female medical'. In those days men and women were always on different wards, and they weren't specialised as now. If a woman was admitted with a medical condition she would automatically go to a female medical ward. If she was coming in for an operation it would be a female surgical ward.

This left male medical and, last but not least, male surgical ward, which was the most popular with the cadet nurses. Surgical patients were a lot younger, which inevitably meant there was friendly banter on the wards. The men didn't seem to complain as much as the women. Or so it seemed to us cadet nurses.

Each morning I would get off the bus on the corner of Heath Street, which was the road that ran alongside the hospital. There was wasteland on the left side of the street – the houses had been completely demolished and it was fast becoming the local rubbish tip. On the right side there were about 30 dilapidated terraced houses; some of them boarded up with galvanised steel, while others appeared to have people living in them. It was a long road and on the corner there was an old pub.

I usually arranged to meet my friend Patsy on the bus and we'd walk down Heath Street together. We felt safer in twos, and we felt vulnerable if we ever had to walk down that street on our own.

We were usually laughing and joking about all types of things. I remember feeling quite envious of Patsy as she was working on a male surgical ward, but at least she had some funny stories to tell me. Most of the time we were in our own little world and not really paying much attention to what was actually happening around us.

One particular morning there was a woman standing at her window and looking out. Her house was about halfway down the street. The reason I remember it so well was because she seemed to be in a trance, just staring at us.

She looked really scary. Her hair had been dyed black at some point but her roots were very noticeable and it looked like she hadn't brushed it in months. She was wearing an old candlewick dressing gown, with a mug (of tea, I assumed) in one hand and a cigarette in the other.

It was very unusual to see anyone who lived in that street awake early in the morning, so perhaps that was another reason why we noticed her at the window. Patsy joked, 'Look at that woman staring at you. Are you sure she's not a long-lost relative? Come to think of it, she does look a bit like you!' I remember giving her a friendly nudge and we were both giggling as we hurried along the street.

The second thing happened at the end of July 1973, when I was delighted at the thought of breaking up for two weeks' holiday. I arranged to meet Patsy at the end of our shift and we walked through the hospital grounds together linking arms, as we so often did. Then at exactly the same time we took a deep breath and a little skip and shouted, 'Yes, fresh air and we're on holiday for a whole two weeks!' It was a lovely summer's day and the sun was still shining, even though it was late afternoon.

We decided to go for a walk in Summerfield Park which, is at the far end of Dudley Road. We sat there chatting, comparing our stories from the wards, before realising that we had lost all track of time. We hurried along Dudley Road as we were both conscious that we were going to be in serious trouble for getting home so late.

We noticed a few chairs had been placed on the pavement outside the pub on the corner of Heath Street as it was still very warm. A drunk Irishwoman sat on one of the chairs with a pint of cider in her hand. Two men, also the worse for drink, were sitting either side of her with pints of beer in their hands, leering. As 17-year-old girls we were feeling really scared and uncomfortable because of the two men's unwanted glances.

Patsy whispered, 'Why are they looking at us in that pervy way?' I said we should just ignore them.

One of the men suddenly stood up and almost fell over at the same time. He just about managed to save his dignity and steadied himself, then hesitated as if he was about to come towards us. Changing his mind, he started shouting in a strong Dublin accent, his voice slurred and his manner intimidating, 'These are the posh birds that work at the hospital. They won't look at the likes of me.'

Then, with his hand shaking and his other hand

steadying his index finger, he pointed at himself as if to ensure we had no doubt who he was actually referring to. 'No,' he continued, 'we wouldn't be good enough for 'em.'

The second man who was sitting in the other chair was laughing, then he suddenly shouted, 'Are you both still virgins? Only we can soon put that right.'

We became even more anxious and were desperate to get away. By now they were all laughing as if they all thought it was one big joke. All of them were very drunk and had probably been drinking for most of the day. It was before the licensing laws had changed, so I'm sure they'd been drinking heavily before even going to the pub.

Patsy grabbed my arm and shouted, 'Come on, Phyllis, your mum will be wondering where you are.'

Looking back, I now wonder, could that possibly have been my birth mother sitting on the chair between those two drunken men, laughing about crude remarks being made to two young, innocent girls? We both started to run along Heath Street as fast as we could, terrified of the two drunk men and upset by their lewd comments.

We were relieved when the bus arrived almost straightaway. From that day we always referred to that pub as 'the dirty old man's pub'. We avoided walking past, especially if it was a sunny day and there were going to be drunks sitting outside.

It was only when writing this book that these two incidents came back to me so very clearly. I am now certain that it was my mother I saw both times.

Although I think every child deserves to know the truth about their birth parents, they also need to be told in the right way. To have found out that my birth mother was a down-and-out and a chronic alcoholic at such an impressionable age could well have done more harm than good.

I remember when Patsy shouted my name, the drunken woman looked towards me. She did appear troubled in some way, as if she was in deep thought, or maybe she was just too drunk even to have noticed. I've often thought to myself that perhaps, when she was sober, and had had time to reflect on what had actually happened that day, she may have realised that she too had a daughter called Phyllis whom she had left at the orphanage more than 16 years before.

But for me, then, it was paramount that I concentrated on my studies to enable me to qualify as a nurse.

If I had met my alcoholic mother then, it would have changed my life, and I fear not for the better.

It was now May 1974 and I was heading for my eighteenth birthday. I'd arranged to go out for a few drinks with some friends but it certainly wasn't going to be in the type of pub my mother frequented. I always thought of her on my birthday, and wondered if she was thinking about me.

I completed my cadet nurse's course, and on 4 July 1974, I started my nurse training. It was American Independence Day, and I remember thinking it was an appropriate date to move into the nurses' home.

I was at last independent and also very relieved that I wouldn't again have to walk along Heath Street. The nurses' home was situated at the back of the hospital, and the bus stop was outside – buses went straight into the city centre in the opposite direction to Heath Street. Obviously, at the time I had no idea that in fact it was my own mother who I was trying to avoid.

I threw myself into my hospital training and relished being well on the way to becoming a fully qualified nurse. I can still conjure up the plastic swing doors which led to the traditional Nightingale wards and never seemed to close properly; the long, echoing corridors and the old fashioned lifts with metal criss-cross gates that were squeaky and heavy as you heaved them open and shut.

I also absolutely loved being a young 18-year-old, living away from home. Some nights we went out to pubs and sometimes we played music having a girly night in. I was starting to enjoy myself, although I was always aware about not getting too close to the boys – I didn't want to get pregnant.

Five of us from the course went on a trip to Jersey, a first girly holiday! I was able to be bubbly without the fear of being told off. But it was also important to me to study hard and get on. I was conscious of being respectable and getting things right, and I was always level-headed.

At that time I drifted apart from my adoptive mother. Only Dad came to see me at the nurses' home. He came to look over my first car, which I was buying from a ward sister, and he came up to the ward and looked so proud of me in my uniform. I just visited Mum on Boxing Day with the rest of the family and on her birthday.

***

There was another significant incident when I was a year into my training and working in the Accident and Emergency Department. My placement was for eight weeks, enabling me to gain experience in critical care. It wasn't somewhere that I really enjoyed working, mainly because some of the trained staff could be quite intimidating. It could be frantically busy and often very scary. You had to think on your feet; at times it was a matter of life or death.

There was a particular Irish staff nurse who worked in the department. She was referred to by the students as 'The Battle Axe', and she was a real bully who didn't have any time for those still learning. It was as if she had forgotten that she was once a student herself, and she had no patience.

One morning I was unlucky enough to be working on the same shift as her. I heard her talking to one of the junior doctors who was complaining that, 'I can never find anything in this department.' I'm sure he didn't mean anything by his comment and was probably just having a general moan, but the staff nurse immediately became defensive and shouted, 'That's the bloody student nurses for you. They're always putting things back in the wrong place.' Before he could even respond she continued, 'Why the hell we have them on such a busy department, God only knows.' I was a nervous wreck if ever I had to work on her shift and I never learnt a thing. I was determined that when I qualified I would never treat a student in such a way.

If you worked a Saturday late shift it was inevitable that you would be dealing with the local drunks. They had often been fighting and needed attention for their cuts and bruises. Usually arrested by the police for being drunk and disorderly, they were very loud and disruptive, shouting abuse at us.

When you were sitting in the staff room you would sometimes overhear the doctors and nurses complaining about the problems the drunks were causing within the department – you'd hear, 'I wish they would get their lives sorted out as they are costing the NHS so much time and money.' The feeling was that we should be looking after really ill people who deserved our help, as that was what we trained for.

Although understanding their point of view, I always had a degree of sympathy and felt empathy towards vulnerable people, especially when they had some type of addiction. After all, alcoholism is an illness and, as health professionals, we should be there to help everyone.

Another frustration about working in A & E was that you never got to know the patients. When they were brought in they were normally taken straight into a cubicle and then, if they needed to be admitted, a porter and a nurse would escort them on to the ward.

The patients were often referred to as cubicle numbers instead of by their names, and you didn't get to know them as individuals and were usually left wondering how they were getting on.

I was working a 12-hour shift one Saturday. It was June 1975, and I had desperately wanted to change with another student nurse so I could have the day off, but I knew it would be almost impossible. Saturday was not a popular day to work, let alone having to work for 12 hours, so reluctantly I had to do the shift after celebrating Patsy's nineteenth birthday on the Friday night. I certainly wasn't firing on all cylinders.

I arrived on duty that morning at 7.30 a.m., feeling hung-over from the previous night's celebrations. To make matters even worse the Battle Axe was in charge of the department on that particular day. This of course added to the agony of having to work the shift that I would never forget.

When handing over to the day staff, the night staff

said that a 47-year-old woman called Bridget had been brought in around 2 a.m. by the police. Of course, the name meant nothing to me at the time, as I didn't know my birth mother's Christian name. She had been arrested for being drunk and disorderly and was involved in some type of disturbance in the local pub. They had said she was 'a known alcoholic and lived in the area'. The police were concerned about a cut on her forehead, which was deep and had bled a lot.

She had been taken to one of the cubicles and I could hear her shouting and swearing in a strong Irish accent. She was very loud and was making my hang-over even worse.

Her face was swollen and badly bruised with a mixture of congealed blood and eye make-up on each cheek. I noticed a tatty-looking pair of sandals hanging over the trolley. The rest of her was covered by a blanket.

The look of trust in her eyes strangely moved me, as she determinedly clung to the bed's stainless steel safety sides. In my hung-over state I wondered, How on earth can anyone feel like this all the time? I was a student nurse and only into the second week of my placement, and I hadn't had a lot of experience in dealing with drunken, aggressive patients. The whole thing was daunting, to say the least.

I tried to give her some reassurance but she wasn't listening. She started to throw her arms around and at one point, almost punched me in the face. Eventually I managed to calm her down and give her a wash. She had wet herself and needed to be made comfortable, and with a bit of a struggle I managed to put a clean nightdress on her. She did appear to be more settled and lay down and was soon fast asleep. I was then sent on a coffee break.

On my return the Battle Axe shouted at me, so that everyone could hear, and I wished the ground would swallow me up – 'Nurse Price, can you wake up? Whatever is the matter with you this morning? Get the woman in cubicle two a vomit bowl unless you want to have to clean her up again.'

As I turned my head away she shouted, 'Come back. Don't you realise that if someone has been drinking to excess, you must always put them in the recovery position? They could easily inhale their own vomit, which could cause them to aspirate and possibly choke. Then young lady, you would certainly be in a lot of trouble, and would you really want that on your conscience?'

To think I could have been responsible for my own mother choking!

I felt like I was in the middle of a major operation and couldn't get away from the Battle Axe quickly enough, so I ran to the sluice, only to be reprimanded again.

'How many times have I had to tell you not to run in the department?'

I was so nervous I couldn't even find one vomit bowl in the sluice. They were normally always piled up in the corner, but today of all days there were none to be seen. I felt like I was having a panic attack. My heart was racing and I was sweating profusely. I felt in need of a vomit bowl myself. I tried to calm down and took a few slow deep breaths. After a few minutes I went back to face the music.

Back in cubicle two, I discovered that the Irish patient wasn't vomiting and there was certainly nothing wrong with her vocal cords. The staff nurse appeared to have mellowed slightly when I went back and she was singing, 'It's a long way to Tipperary; it's a long way to go' with Bridget. I even heard her talking about me in a jovial way, 'I think Nurse Price has actually gone to Tipperary for that vomit bowl, don't you?' At the time I just thought it was her attempt at trying to be sarcastic, but much later I realised that the staff nurse was also Irish and had probably recognised Bridget's Tipperary accent.

I was sent on my lunch break. I am sure she was losing patience with me and just wanted me out of the way. When I returned there was already another patient in cubicle two and I remember feeling relieved as it was so much quieter. All I wanted to do was finish my shift without getting into any more trouble.

When I first met my mother six years later, and heard her distinctive Tipperary accent and saw her bruised and swollen face, I had a flashback to the woman in cubicle two and realised that my mother was indeed that disruptive drunk. To think she had no idea that I was the daughter she had left at the orphanage many years before. It is upsetting to think that possibly one of the worst days I can ever remember in my nursing career, when I really did need some moral support, my own mother was actually there in cubicle two. She was the woman who nearly choked on her own vomit because of my inexperience of dealing with drunken patients.

***

By August 1975 I had finished my placement in A & E and was only too glad to be seeing the back of the Battle Axe. To my surprise she actually gave me a good report, but during the rest of my nurse training I had very little involvement with any of the local drunks and avoided the pubs where they hung out.

As I've mentioned before, I wasn't really thinking a lot about my adoption at this time. I was happy, busy studying, and mostly enjoying my placements.

My favourite had been the male surgical ward, especially as I was working with one of my closest friends, Helen. The sister was lovely and she often commented how we brought such laughter to her ward – although at times it also got us into trouble and she would have to separate us, as we got fits of the giggles with the patients.

That in itself could cause problems. The men were usually recovering from some form of abdominal surgery and had stitches, and in those days there were no clips or glue to hold the wound together. Many a time I remember them holding their stomachs and telling us to stop making them laugh as their stitches could burst open. Working on this ward was so much fun. Obviously some of the patients were extremely poorly, but as they started to recover we would do our best to cheer them up.

On one occasion, when I was doing my medication assessment, I asked one of the older patients, who was a little hard of hearing, 'Have you had your bowels open today?' Still not understanding what I had said, I showed him this chart where it said 'B/O'.

He rather abruptly replied, 'I haven't got body odour. I had a shower this morning.'

The man in the next bed behind the curtains shouted, 'Bill, stop making such a fuss. She only wants to know if you've had a shit this morning.'

'Well why didn't she ask me that in the first place?' he replied. I ended up with a terrible fit of the giggles.

After completing my training, and working on the new geriatric unit at Dudley Road for nine months, I decided that I needed a change and wanted to gain more experience in another area of nursing. So, early in 1978, I enrolled on a post-natal and neo-natal course for nine months at Sorrento Maternity Hospital in Moseley.

As I was leaving Dudley Road Hospital, I also had to move out of the nurses' home, which meant moving back to live with my adoptive parents as there was no nurses' accommodation at Sorrento Hospital.

Carole had got married in 1977. She and her husband had bought an old house, and they lived at Mum's while doing it up. When I came home, carrying my boxes, Mum told me not to disturb Carole's husband as he was watching the football in the living room.

I said, 'Oh, well I'll just pop my head round the door to say hello.' But was told, 'No, no, you go straight upstairs.' As I walked up to my room, I remember thinking, Nothing's changed here.

As I was on a course I didn't have to work shifts, so I was able to drive myself to work each morning. It is strange, but although I hadn't even started to try to trace my birth mother at that point, it was as if in some way we were always drawn to each other, without either of us realising it.

Unbelievably, for the second time I had to pass by my mother's house – this time in Balsall Heath, where she would have been living then. Thankfully, I was now in a car and obviously not so vulnerable when driving past what was probably her local pub.

In the afternoon, I usually drove home to Erdington a different way so that I could give my friend a lift home. She sometimes said she felt awful making my journey home so much longer. I always reassured her that it was a much nicer area to drive through and that there were often strange-looking people lurking about in the Balsall Heath area.

By October 1978 I had started working as a district nurse, which is what I had dreamt of doing since talking to Mrs Brewin as a young girl. I always hoped that one day I would be able to do the same job as the district nurse who visited her husband.

I remember she would save newspapers for the nurses, and as a young girl I used to think to myself that they couldn't be very busy if they had time to be reading the newspaper all day. As a district nurse myself now, working in Stechford in Birmingham, and in Sandwell, I realised that the newspapers were needed to put on the floor when removing soiled bandages. We were always very busy, and certainly didn't have time to read newspapers! But I soon discovered that I had made the right choice in my career path and had great job satisfaction from it. And it helped me so much when I was finally able to meet my mother.

Chapter 6

The Search Begins

I met Stephen on 17 February 1976. My friend Christine and I had just given blood and we decided we'd go out for once – after all, the staff had said to drink plenty of fluids (of course, they didn't mean the fluids we had in mind).

It was a Tuesday night, so after going to a couple of pubs in Birmingham we ended up at the Party Night at the Cedar Club. Everyone was flirting with everyone else and having a great time. The disc jockey said, 'Ladies, turn to the man on your right and ask him what colour underpants he's got on?' So I turned – and Stephen was standing there – I asked him what colour he was wearing, and noticed he had a nice smile. So, when the DJ said, 'Grab a partner,' I grabbed him and took him up on stage. There were six couples, and we stood facing each other with a balloon between us. The first couple to put a T-shirt on over the top won a bottle of champagne. Stephen and I won!

We sat down with Christine and her man. Christine was smoking, and Stephen was staring at me, as if weighing me up, waiting for me to do something. I said, 'I don't smoke, you know.'

'Oh that's good,' he replied. 'If you did smoke I wouldn't go out with you.'

'What makes you think I want to go out with you anyway?' I answered back.

We both knew there was an attraction as we went for a taxi later. We arranged to meet a couple of nights after outside Rackham's. I still have my blood card and the champagne cork from that day.

It became a serious relationship and after two years we decided to tie the knot. Stephen was dependable and caring. We loved each other, but I also felt secure and thought he'd be a good father. I wanted to be part of a normal family, married with my own children. And with Stephen I knew we had a mature relationship.

He was on my side too. When Mum couldn't come to the engagement party and Carole started making excuses, he was happy to say, 'Let's not worry about them, let's go out for a meal, just us.'

***

I hadn't told anyone I was adopted since primary school, and it was when I was busy arranging the wedding in May 1979 that I suddenly realised I hadn't even told Stephen.

When you get married in a Catholic church, the parish priest needs proof that you have been baptised into that faith. This would normally be a simple enough thing to do but, unsurprisingly, when I asked my adoptive mother for my baptismal certificate she almost had a nervous breakdown. She told me the certificate had been 'lost', but that it was nothing for me to worry about and that she would sort it out with the priest.

Instead, my adoptive mother hurried along to the church to give the priest the certificate without my knowledge. What gave her the right to deny me that information about myself?

I tried asking her a few questions about it, how old I was when I was baptised, in which church, and she became very annoyed, bellowing, 'I knew you were going to be asking too many questions. Will you ever be grateful for what we have done for you? We took you out of the orphanage and gave you a better life, and still you're not satisfied.'

She really was missing the point. I wasn't questioning how they had treated me as adoptive parents, it was just a simple question, but she had told so many lies about the circumstances around my adoption and she was terrified that the truth would one day come out.

I really wanted to find out about my origins because I wanted to have a child of my own. I needed to know if there were any hereditary health problems, but in any case it was my human right to be told the truth about my origins. But until I was an adult and took control, it was something I was always denied.

She didn't even allow me to see the baptismal certificate. In 2010 I received my adoption papers and it was amongst them. Thirty years after my marriage I did finally get to see it.

Of course, I had never been allowed to be open about my adoption, and I almost lived in fear of it becoming public. Then, a few weeks before my wedding, I blurted it out to Stephen. His reaction was surprisingly matter of fact, and I soon realised that it was fine to tell people. It was not a problem! I vividly remember feeling a great sense of relief, the burden I had been carrying with me since my early school years was suddenly lifted. It was a feeling I shall never forget.

I realised that being adopted was not something to be ashamed of. I wasn't a freak, and I wasn't the only person in the world to have been adopted.

We got married a week after my twenty-third birthday, 26 May 1979. It poured down – you couldn't even hear the church bells – but it didn't dampen our day.

We had a week's honeymoon in St Ives and bought a brand new house in Sandwell, a few miles from Stephen's parents in West Bromwich. We were mortgaged up to the hilt, and Mum didn't like that I had a better house than Carole, but we were happy. I also changed districts to work nearer to where I lived.

I felt so liberated, like a bird being let out of a cage and allowed to fly away. I could now start the process of finding out about my true identity. I was no longer living with my adoptive parents, so I wouldn't have to worry when I had any letters through the post about my adoption.

The only document that I was ever allowed to see was the small re-registered birth certificate, the one which made me feel as though I hadn't existed for the four years before I was adopted.

However, when I was about ten years old I found

out that my birth name was Phyllis Larkin. This happened one Saturday afternoon when I was alone in the house with Kevin. He told me about 'Dad's secret suitcase', where he kept all his important papers, and which he always kept locked. I had no idea what he was talking about.

'What papers?' I asked.

His reply was a bolt from the blue. 'Your adoption papers. They're all about when Mum and Dad had to go to court to adopt you.'

He showed me where Dad kept the key in a vase on the mantelpiece. He swore me to secrecy and told me I must never tell a living soul, otherwise he would be in a great deal of trouble. I quickly opened the suitcase. My hands were clammy and shaking, my stomach tightened. I was petrified in case I was caught red-handed. I certainly would have been up against the firing squad.

I nervously lifted the lid of a small shoe box that was in the suitcase, and there in front of my eyes were my adoption papers with my birth name: Phyllis Larkin. I shut the box as quickly as I had opened it and didn't dare go back to those papers ever again. But – what a moment! I actually knew my birth name. It was such a strange feeling.

* * *

About two months after I got married I sent off for my original birth certificate from Somerset House in London. I was given some leaflets and the phone numbers of various support groups. Before I could receive my birth certificate I had to go through a statutory interview with a local social worker called John, who was kind and helpful.

He gave me the usual warnings about tracing my mother. He advised me to be careful and asked me if I was prepared for what I might find.

'Your mother may not even want to meet you,' he warned me. 'It's possible she hasn't told anyone you even exist. She could be married with other children. You really need to prepare yourself for all eventualities. She may have a dysfunctional life, which could be very traumatic for you.'

Little did he know how close he was to the truth, but he soon realised how determined I was, and I was not going to change my mind. I explained how I hadn't been given any information from my adoptive parents about the reasons why I was put up for adoption. He seemed shocked, particularly when I said I was told that both my parents had died. He reassured me that he would do his best to help. We arranged a second meeting a few weeks later. By this time, he had received my birth certificate and could give me some information about who I really was.

I glanced nervously over his desk and could see my birth certificate in front of him.

'Your mother was called Bridget Larkin,' he said.

Of course I already knew her surname was Larkin, but I hadn't told him about my dad's secret suitcase. It had her address as Bryon Street in Coventry, and in the space for listing occupation, it said that she was a waitress for a motor company. My father was 'unknown', which didn't come as any surprise. I'd always felt that she must have been an unmarried mother, and that that was the main reason she'd had me adopted.

As an adopted person every little detail is so important to you. I had been denied this information all my life, and now there it was in front of me. This was the first time I had heard my mother's name. All her life people had called her Bridget and I never knew. This may sound trivial, but what you have to remember is that from a very early age almost everyone knows their mother's Christian name. If you are fortunate to have your mother bring you up, then you will constantly hear relatives and friends calling her by that name. When you meet someone for the first time, one of the first questions you usually ask is their name. Yet I was 23 years old before I ever knew my own mother's name.

The next meeting I had with John was in October 1979. He told me, 'Now you've had a chance to get used to the details about your mother, the next thing we need to do is try and find out where she is living now.' The address on my birth certificate was the first lead, but I told John I had already driven to that address in Coventry and the houses had long since been demolished.

John looked shocked. He emphasised to me the importance of not going it alone. He asked, 'What on earth would you have done if your mother was living at that address and she had come to the door?'

I felt rather told off. I hadn't given it a great deal of thought, I suppose. I had just been impatient, but I realised he was right. I reassured him that in future I would not try to do things by myself.

The next step would be to check the electoral register; and he also asked me the name of the orphanage. John said he would be in touch when he had any more information.

He could see how much it meant to me, and said he was going to do his best to help me trace my mother.

A few days later he phoned with some surprising news. John had contacted Father Hudson's Homes and to his amazement a woman called May McFadden, who had actually helped arrange my adoption, was still working there. She had been at the orphanage for more than 30 years. She told John that she remembered me and my mother well and was more than happy to arrange a meeting at the orphanage.

It was very emotional returning all those years later. My memories came flooding back. Stephen drove me and waited for me in the car, and as I walked up to the front entrance it looked exactly the same as when I was there all those years ago.

I walked through the main reception area and there were the almost clinical chequered black-and-white tiles. The place still smelt the same: a general mustiness, partly disguised by a strong smell of wax polish. I told myself it was imperative that my emotions were put to one side. I had to be strong, or at least appear that way.

The meeting was surprisingly formal. May McFadden introduced herself to me and explained her role within the orphanage. There was no affectionate embrace or reassuring smile to help put me at my ease.

Miss McFadden explained how the orphanage had been run then. Canon Flynn had been in charge and organised all the adoptions with the help of the Mother Superior, Sister Bernadette. 'I was top management, you know,' said Miss McFadden, as if in some way trying to impress me. 'I had to make a lot of very important decisions about the babies' futures.'

Her role in the orphanage had been like that of a social worker, as back in those days things were very much kept within the locked doors of the orphanage. The most important criteria would be to find what they called 'a good Catholic family'. Prospective parents would need to be married for at least nine months, just to make sure to the outside world that everything appeared respectable. If they were Catholic and married they must be good! Obviously this was not always the case.

I didn't warm to Miss McFadden in the slightest. She had a really authoritarian manner, showed little compassion, and seemed determined to prevent me from meeting my mother. She ensured that she remained in total control for the entire meeting, and even commented how well I had been brought up. How she came to that conclusion I'm a little unsure, as she hadn't even asked me one question about my life after I left the orphanage.

This was not the time to have told her that, as a child, things were not always good, and I didn't dare question her decisions. Instead, I listened attentively to what she had decided to tell me. I didn't have any recollection of her when I was at the orphanage, I'm pleased to say. She told me that 'most of her time was spent in the offices sorting out the adoptions.' She appeared to have little time for the children, which was probably for the best. She hadn't married and made it quite clear she had never wanted children of her own.

At this point we had a break for a much-needed cup of tea, although I could have done with something much stronger, under the circumstances. Next she showed me around the orphanage, which I found extremely emotional. Part of it had been closed off, but inside the home it still resembled a church, a place to worship instead of somewhere you could call home. It had a strong smell of old wood, but it had been kept nice and clean. There was a large crucifix in the main entrance hall. In my head, I could hear the sounds of us children singing grace before our meals, usually out of time and with no real thought of what we were actually praying about. I'm sure we were just hoping to be allowed to sit down and eat.

I was aware of the importance of not upsetting Miss McFadden, so intermittently I gave her a false smile, trying my best not to antagonise her. It felt like I had come for an interview to get a job, for which I feared I may not have even been shortlisted by the look on her face. I reminded myself the main reason why I was here in the first place, not that it was something I was ever likely to forget.

It was 1979 and there were now fewer children to be adopted as, thankfully, the stigma of having a child out of wedlock had almost disappeared. I was led upstairs into the nursery, still having to patiently await any information about my mother. It was as if she was trying to rub salt into my wounds, showing me how little and fragile I must have been when my mother first left me. As we walked into the nursery the babies were all fast asleep in their cots.

She looked at them and said, 'I really find it hard to comprehend how any mother could ever leave their baby here.' That was the last thing I needed to hear.

By now I had tears running down my face, which was something I was desperately trying to avoid. She almost seemed pleased that I was upset, maybe secretly hoping I might then show some anger towards my mother for leaving me at the orphanage in the first place. That was something I was determined not to show, at least not in front of someone who was so judgemental. But I felt upset at the thought of having to be left as a baby, and couldn't begin to imagine how my mother must have felt leaving me in the nursery all those years ago.

I asked her, 'Was this the actual nursery where I would have stayed?' and she replied in an almost dismissive manner, 'Yes, this is where all the baby girls stayed until they were twelve months old.' Desperate for answers I continued, 'Would my mother have come into this nursery?' With a sarcastic frown she replied, 'Yes, on the rare occasions she could be bothered to visit.' It was obvious that she had little time for my mother and was doing everything in her power to persuade me to be of the same opinion.

This was the place my mother had had to part with me. I tried not to dwell on that too much as I was already feeling very emotional about the whole experience. There were six cots in the nursery and the only thing to identify the babies was a tag at the end of their cots with their surname written on in capital letters. This was a very moving encounter; it was the last bit of the babies' true identity they had left. I asked, 'Will the babies be told their original surname?'

She replied abruptly, 'Of course not. They will have a new surname when they are adopted and that is the only name they will need to know.' By this time I sensed she had detached herself from the whole situation and appeared to show little, if any, emotion. I started to feel very angry inside and wanted to shout, That is something they might want to know, the last bit of their true identity, and they have a right to know. But my mouth went dry and no words came out, so my thoughts remained unsaid.

When I was standing in the nursery I was drawn to a baby in the corner. The tag said 'Kelly' and it was pink, so I knew then that the baby was a little girl. She was lovely. I so wanted to pick her up and give her a cuddle. She had a mop of ginger hair and spots over her face, maybe a milk rash which a lot of babies get. Who knows, Kelly may even have children of her own by now. I do hope she had a happy childhood.

My emotions were all over the place and I asked Miss

McFadden if I could hold the baby. 'No,' she shouted, 'visitors are not allowed to pick up the babies. They will be placed for adoption by the time they are six weeks old.' She was so dismissive. It was as if the babies were on a conveyor belt, waiting to be picked by a respectable Catholic married couple looking for a child to adopt. I was caught up with the moment and asked, 'Can I adopt baby Kelly?' Instead of reassuring me that the little baby girl would be going to a loving home, I was told abruptly, 'Just because you have been adopted doesn't give you the right to adopt. Surely you want your own children? A baby that will resemble you.' She had taken what I said literally, instead of understanding that I was just getting a little bit carried away with what I was experiencing.

Again I realised that I needed to detach myself from any emotions. I wanted to find out about my mother, and had to be strong and stay focused on what I had come to do, so I allowed her to remain in control. The fact that she had not considered my feelings about being adopted was something I needed to forget. She still had vital information which she hadn't given me, and the last thing I wanted to do was annoy her in any way, because she had the power to withhold it. She appeared as if she was becoming a little impatient with my questions.

She suddenly said, 'Let's go back downstairs to my office.' She ushered me in saying, 'Come along now, sit down, the chair's not going to bite you.' And off she went to find my adoption file. It felt as if she had been gone for ages but it was probably only a few minutes. I started to feel annoyed – surely my file should have been ready, as she'd been expecting me? She was determined to stay in control and I had to remind myself that she was good enough to take the time to see me in the first place, albeit on her terms. I knew what I was about to hear wasn't going to be good, but I yearned to know everything, warts and all.

I could never have prepared myself for what she told me about my mother. She started to explain that my mother first contacted Father Hudson's Homes through a social worker based in Coventry, as she was finding it hard to cope. She said, 'Your mother decided to leave you at the orphanage when you were just eight months old. She honestly believed that she would be able to come back to collect you when her life got back on track, which obviously never happened.'

When my mother took me into the orphanage in January 1957 it was extremely cold; she was finding it hard to look after a baby by herself, and worried about paying her heating bill. Apparently I was a really bonny baby; in fact a little bit on the fat side.

'I'd say your mother had tried to do her best to look after you by herself. All your clothes were brought in clean and in good condition,' said Miss McFadden. For a short time she actually seemed quite sympathetic towards her. I felt quite touched by how my mother had cared for me for the first eight months of my life, and how she had struggled to look after me by herself.

Miss McFadden swiftly started explaining how my mother would write for a pass, which is what the orphanage had to ask the mothers to do if they wanted to visit their babies. She said, 'Your mother would often ask for the pass and then just not turn up, presumably drunk from the previous night. It's a blessing you were so young and weren't able to understand, otherwise you would have been so disappointed.' I could tell by her voice that it irritated her.

Although in theory I agreed with what she was saying, I was determined not to dwell on anything negative at that point. I wanted to hear the whole story first before I came to any conclusions.

I asked about my father. Had my mother known him

for long? In what I can only recall as a rather matter-of-fact reply to such a sensitive question she said with a disapproving expression on her face, 'Well …' She paused for a few moments before taking a slow deep breath and putting her hand under her chin.

'Regarding your father, I can't tell you very much because, not surprisingly, your mother didn't tell us very much. She told us she met him in a night club in Hurst Street in Birmingham. Your mother didn't know his name, but told us that she would recognise him again if she saw him.' Looking puzzled she continued, 'Although that would be highly unlikely, according to your mother.' With that information it seemed pretty obvious that I wasn't conceived out of love.

I told myself there may be more I could find out about my father. Perhaps my mother had lied to the nuns about him because she needed to leave me at the orphanage, and if she had told them she had any contact with him it would just have complicated things.

I also realised she was withholding vital information that, in her opinion, was better I didn't hear. She was being very secretive and I felt extremely frustrated. There was my file across the table, which I felt I had a right to read. I longed to see the file for myself. At one point I leant over to try and get just a glimpse of what had been written about me, I was so desperate for every minute detail. She just looked across the table with a very grim face, peering over her glasses and slammed my file shut. She didn't have to say a word.

So I knew the questions to ask without causing her to become irritated any further. I tried to convince her that I didn't approve of the lifestyle my mother was leading. I sensed that if she thought that I was going to be influenced or sympathetic towards my mother she wouldn't have told me as much, maybe wrongly thinking that I would meet up with her and be led astray by her dysfunctional lifestyle. I knew that would never happen – by now I was a mature person in my own right, and certainly would never have wanted to live the life that my mother was living.

Neither was I there to judge her. I was very level-headed, had given tracing my mother a lot of thought and I had prepared myself for any eventualities. She seemed a little more at ease about giving me the information on my file and suddenly started to tell me the hard facts. Maybe she realised how determined I was to find out as much as I could.

'Your mother was a bit of a one and liked the good

life,' she said. Sadly a good life was something she never had, I thought. 'She never seemed to learn from her mistakes.'

I told myself that I was not going to be influenced by her prejudices; this was my mother not hers, my own flesh and blood. My mother was vulnerable and it sounded to me as if she needed a friend or, more importantly, she needed her daughter. I was desperately hoping that it was not too late to be able to help her. I was however strongly advised not to contact her. 'I don't think it will help you to go and find her. She has ruined her own life and she will only try to do the same with yours,' said Miss McFadden.

I had to make a promise that I would not try to contact her before she would tell me more. I reassured her of this, crossing my fingers under the table, knowing it was a promise I would certainly not be able to keep. I was sure under the circumstances I'd be forgiven for telling a little white lie.

Maybe if I had been a different type of person I could have walked away and not got involved, but that was never going to happen. She looked at me and said, 'You seem to be taking things well.' If only she really knew how my stomach was churning inside, but I knew that was something I needed to hide from her. It was important that I stayed composed as I wanted as much information as she was prepared to give me. She continually glanced over to study my facial expression and I vaguely remember giving her a half-hearted smile in an attempt to stay in her good books.

She told me how my mother had found it hard to get her life back on track following the birth of her first child, a baby boy called Keiran, whom she had left in an orphanage back in Ireland. This was the first time I knew about my half-brother and, true to form, Miss McFadden allowed me no time to reflect on such a life-changing event. She continued to tell me how my mother was unable to lead a 'normal life' because of her alcohol addiction. It totally ruled her life and was the only thing she really cared about. This was very painful to hear, but it only made me more determined to do my very best to find her and give her all the love she needed.

I felt Miss McFadden did not want me to think about the fact that my mother looked after me by herself for the first eight months of my life. I tried to ask a little bit more about what happened then, but I could hear the annoyance in her voice as she said, quite cruelly, 'Your mother did honestly believe that one day she would just be able to come and collect you. Well, that was when she could be bothered.'

Then I heard an astonishing thing. She told me about a letter my mother had written to the Mother Superior in June 1973. I was so excited and shouted, 'Had she put her address on the letter?'

She paused to put on her glasses. I could hardly contain myself while I waited for her reply. 'Yes, she lived in Heath Street, Winson Green, Birmingham.'

It was an address I knew well. When I was a cadet nurse, in that same year, I must have walked past her house most mornings chatting to my friend Patsy. I suddenly had what I now think was a panic attack. I was sure I must have met my mother before. My head was all over the place and I could hear my heart beating. I took some deep breaths to try to compose myself.

Miss McFadden realised that something was wrong and asked if I was all right. 'Yes,' I replied quickly, although I was anything but. I feared I would have to pay a visit to the confession box if I kept telling all these white lies. I was given a glass of cold water and she opened the window so that I could get some fresh air. At this point she was actually being quite kind, so maybe she did have a heart after all.

But that was not to last. I asked if I could read the letter for myself but she snapped, 'No, it is confidential.'

I felt so annoyed. Then why tell me about it? I thought. At least let me see the letter for myself. This was the one link I had with my mother and I wasn't allowed to read it or even glance at it. Why was I prevented from seeing something that was so personal to me?

I smiled at her, hoping she might change her mind. I said I would love to see my mother's handwriting, to which she replied sarcastically, 'I can tell you it is very scruffy. I think she wrote it in the pub and spilt her drink over it. Her spelling is not too good either.' I couldn't believe how insensitive she was.

By this point I was feeling sick with anger but I knew I had to remain calm. She went on to tell me she thought it was clear that my mother contacted the orphanage only when she realised I was old enough to be a wage-earner, that she wanted 'some money for her booze'.

I'm now convinced that the only reason Miss McFadden had agreed to meet me was in the hope that she would dissuade me from continuing with my search. 'Your mother always believed that she would be able to have you back when her own life did eventually become more stable, but this never happened,' she said. As my mother had not signed the final adoption papers she thought I was still at the orphanage.

This angered Miss McFadden and she shouted, 'Did your mother honestly believe that she could just leave you in limbo at the orphanage until she was good and ready to come and collect you, to deprive you of a loving family and allow you to spend all your childhood in this orphanage? I am sorry to have to say, but it was very selfish of her. Why should she be allowed to play with a child's life like that?'

It was the first time she had shown any real compassion about anything. I did understand what she was upset about and this time she had a valid point, but I was doing my best not to feel any anger towards my mother. I had not even met her yet.

She went on to explain to me that my mother had ignored all correspondence with the orphanage and had been summoned to appear in court so that I could be legally adopted. She failed to turn up on two occasions. Maybe she just could not be bothered, or perhaps it was just too painful. I like to think it was the latter.

Either way, my mother didn't give her written consent for me to be legally adopted, so in her mind I was still waiting to be collected. But it was a hell of a wait. I'm sure my mother had been in denial and just didn't want to get involved with the formalities of the adoption process as it made it too final. Eventually it was taken out of her hands and on the third court hearing the judge overruled the decision. So I was legally adopted and my birth mother was not even aware that it had actually happened.

The orphanage had replied to my mother's 1973 letter, informing her that I had been adopted and they had not heard anything about me for the last 13 years. They told her that as far as adoption goes, no news is good news. I am sure now that my mother got drunk the day she received the letter from the orphanage. It was how she dealt with most of her problems, but it also created so many of them too.

Miss McFadden told me that my mother had often been in trouble with the police, and they were trying to arrange for her to go back to Ireland because of all the problems that she had caused in England. I'm uncertain what the nuns knew about my mother's life when she lived in Ireland, but they knew she was running away from something or someone as she decided to change her surname to Ryan.

Knowing her changed name was an important piece of information, as it eventually led me to her. Without that vital piece of the jigsaw I would never have been able to trace my mother. It was unclear why she was wanted by the police, but by the way Miss McFadden explained it to me, I thought she had probably been a prostitute.

We stopped for a short break and I was taken around the grounds. It brought back such a lot of memories from my childhood. We would spend many sunny afternoons in the garden playing with the nursery nurses, making them pretend cups of tea.

I remembered the wooden balconies around the buildings and the beds being wheeled outside to enable some of the children to enjoy the sunny afternoons while lying down. When I was so young I didn't understand why they stayed in bed all the time. To me they were just being lazy. Even at such a young age I knew not to ask too many questions. The nursery nurses did not usually know the answer and the nuns would just reply, 'You do not need to know that.'

Miss McFadden answered my question all those years later. 'That was the sick bay and the children were often wheeled out in their sick beds as fresh air was thought to be the best medicine.' I felt quite guilty thinking that those poor children were just being lazy and all the time they were ill. At least now I had my question answered, although I'd like to think I'm better at looking after sick people as an adult, especially as I'm a nurse.

We went back into the office and I was aware of the time I had taken, but there was more to be told and I listened attentively. Miss McFadden continued telling me stories about my mother. She supposed that Bridget had tried her best to look after me by herself. 'But she often did not act in a very responsible way. She was lonely, with her nights spent staying in looking after you as a baby.' The nuns worried that on some occasions I had been left by myself as a young baby, though thankfully, I was not harmed in any way. It seemed that my mother was missing her social life and as Miss McFadden continued in her blunt way, 'She was not the brightest and never seemed to use her common sense.' Eventually my mother came to her senses and asked for help, whatever her reasons, and for that I'm extremely grateful.

Miss McFadden checked her watch and appeared a little concerned about the length of time the meeting had taken, but then continued. 'After leaving you at the orphanage your mother very quickly went back to her old ways. She did visit you at first, most Sundays, but she'd often complain that she couldn't afford her travel expenses.'

This apparently annoyed the nuns as she always seemed to find the money to buy alcohol, on which by then she was very dependent. Sometimes when she visited the orphanage she would appear drunk, slurring her words and being very incoherent.

On these visits she would apparently start to lay down the law about the type of adoptive parents she wanted for her daughter. I had to smile about some of the things I was told. Failing that I think I would have been in floods of tears.

At this point I remember Miss McFadden taking a deep breath, and in her assertive manner and high pitched voice shouting, 'Well I do have the rest of the day to get through.' It's a phrase I will never forget as I remember thinking at the time, It's just a polite way of saying, 'I need you to leave now'.

I had received a lot of information, but the day was difficult and very sad. At times I really felt that I was intruding on someone else's life, when in fact it was my life and I had a right to know what actually did happen. Now, as a nurse I often have to care for older people with mental health problems, and one of the things you are taught during your training is not to be judgemental, but to treat people as individuals. So why should that not apply to my own mother? Yes, she had made mistakes, and a few more than most people, but that just made me more determined to try to make contact so that I could care for her.

I was told early in 2010, when I was finally allowed to see my adoption file, that May McFadden had died in a nursing home in 2002 after suffering from dementia for several years. Many people have an impact on our lives, and she would certainly be at the top of my list. I respected her integrity and I am sure in her own strange way she had my best interests at heart. Without her help on that memorable morning in November 1979, I would never have met my birth mother and, though it led me to stormy waters, for that alone I will always be grateful.

Chapter 7

Meeting My Mother

Christmas came and went, and the only thing that seemed important to me at that time was when I would next have a meeting with John. This eventually took place in February 1980. I told John that I had been warned by Miss McFadden to leave well alone, and to get on with the rest of my life. Luckily for me, John was not of the same opinion. In fact he was almost as curious as I was. He said, 'We've come this far. We can't just give up on it now.'

I gave him the two vital pieces of information I had: the name she was using – Bridget Ryan – and her last known address in Winson Green. John reassured me that he would contact me in the week with any information he had.

A few days later he telephoned and said he had only just had some news, but wanted to call me before the weekend. It was a Friday afternoon I will never forget. I could tell by his voice and the way he was hesitating that it was not going to be good news. I tried to prepare myself for what he was about to tell me, but I felt physically sick. I had picked up the phone in the bedroom, and now I sat down on the bed as I was shaking and dreaded to hear whatever was coming.

He had contacted the General Hospital in Birmingham, as he felt they may have known Bridget. Sure enough he was right. They knew her well.

'Two years ago your mother was admitted into hospital in a bad state, with a fractured femur. She was a well-known alcoholic in the area and had been very ill indeed. She had been in and out of the A & E department on many occasions, but she hadn't been seen since.'

Then came the bombshell.

'Those who saw her in the hospital thought it unlikely that she could survive another two years in her condition,' he said, and then paused, floundering a little. He knew that he was about to tell me the one thing I was dreading to hear.

'I'm sorry, but I think you had better assume that she is dead. Maybe I could help you to find out where she is buried?'

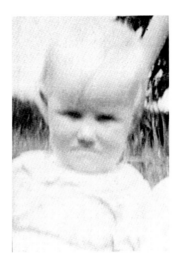
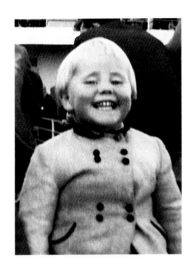

Above left: Phyllis as a baby at the orphanage.
Right: On a boat, her first outing after leaving the orphanage to start a new life.
Below left: At church, aged six, wishing she had a veil instead of a hat.
Right: Phyllis at school, at the age of seven, around the time she told a friend the secret of her adoption.

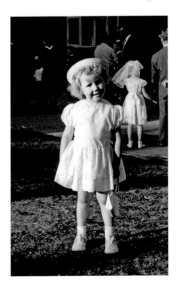
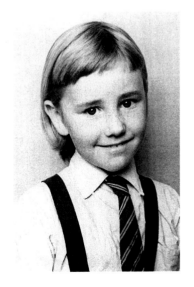

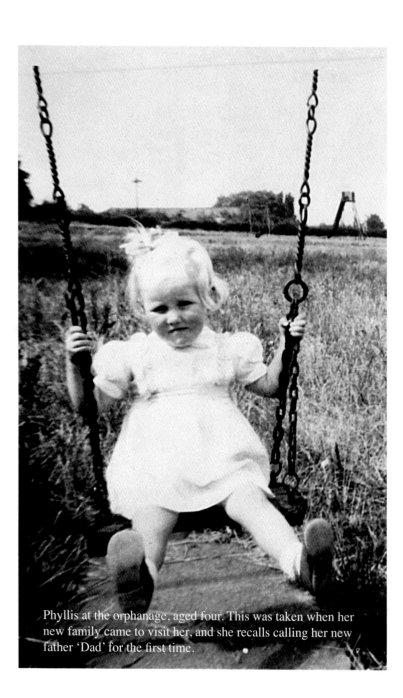

Phyllis at the orphanage, aged four. This was taken when her new family came to visit her, and she recalls calling her new father 'Dad' for the first time.

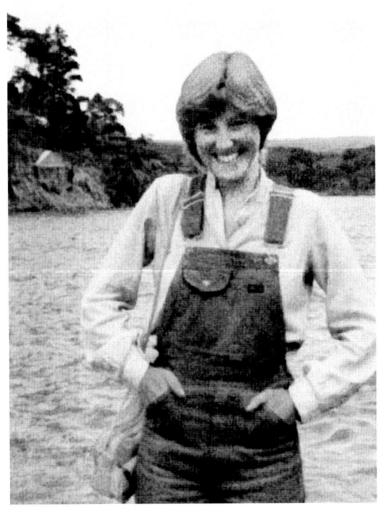

Phyllis at the age of 23, when she took the momentous decision to begin the search for her birth mother.

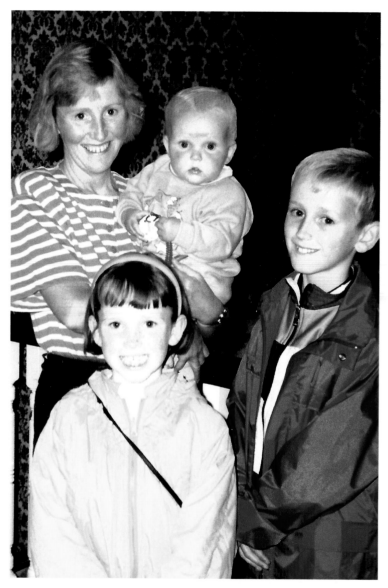

Phyllis with her children, Tom (8 months), Stuart (10) and Hannah (7). Less than a year later, Tom went to the nursing home to meet his grandmother.

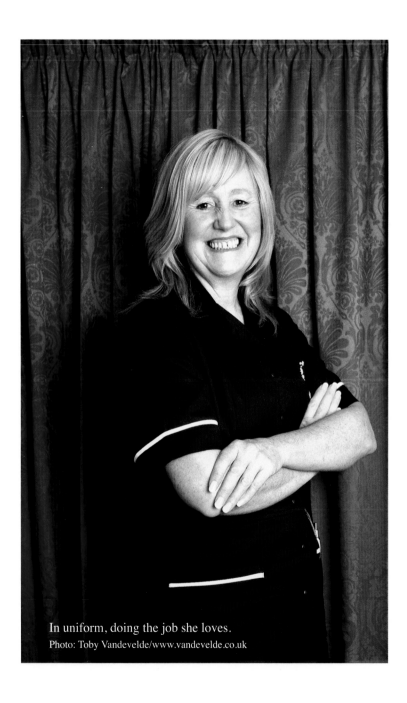

In uniform, doing the job she loves.
Photo: Toby Vandevelde/www.vandevelde.co.uk

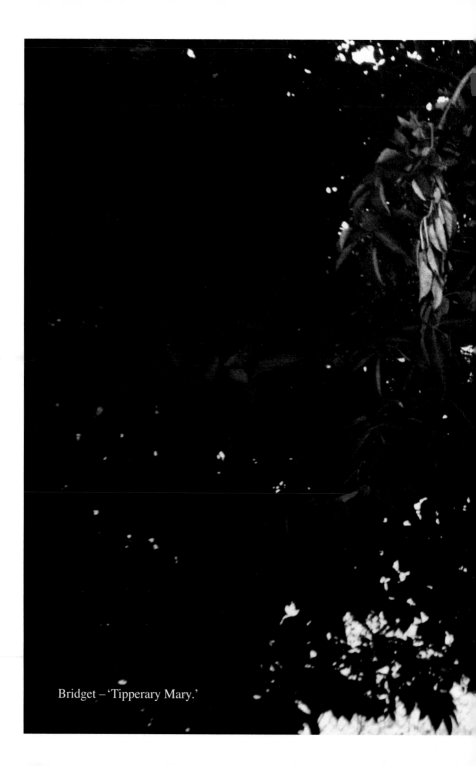

Bridget – 'Tipperary Mary.'

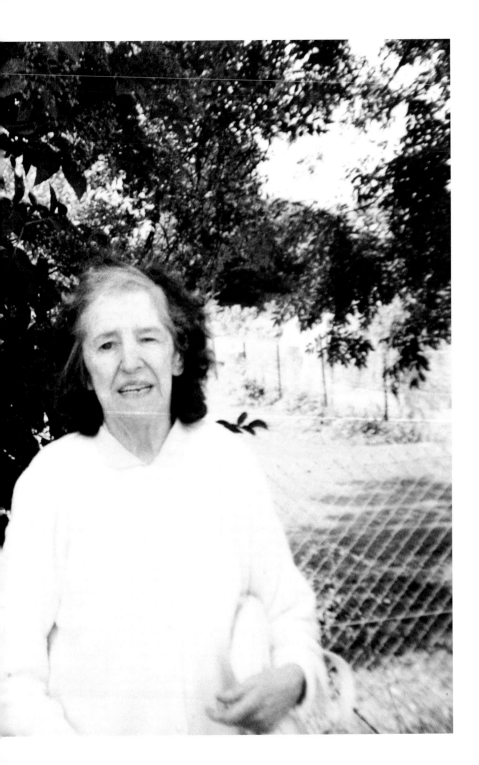

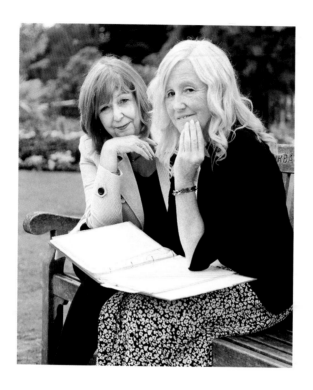

Phyllis, with her friend and co-author, Barbara Fisher, and at home in Birmingham.

Photos: Roy Edwards

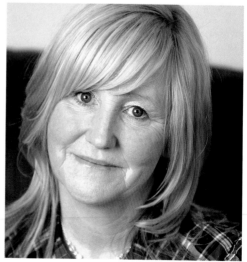

I suppose it was all I could have hoped for under the circumstances. I felt numb, but I heard myself uttering a few pleasantries, mainly thanking him for his time in trying to help trace her. I think it was my attempt to be discreet, and to avoid exposing my true feelings. I did not want to take out my anger on the one person who had at least tried to help me trace my mother. I burst into tears as I put down the phone.

It was such an anti-climax. Why was I crying for someone I didn't even know? But this was my mother, my own flesh and blood. I would never now have the chance to meet her. It just seemed so cruel. There were so many unanswered questions spinning around in my head: had she died alone and full of regrets? Had she died a terrible alcoholic death, choking on her own vomit, lying in a gutter somewhere, with nobody to care for her?

But there was nobody to answer any of them. I would never be able to tell her that she did the right thing when she gave me up for adoption. I wanted to tell her that I was now a nurse, and perhaps I could have been able to look after her and given her some love, which she had been denied all her life. Maybe I could have taken some of her pain and guilt away. I already knew a great deal about her, but what did she look like? I would never be able to find out. Why had I left it so long before I tried to trace her? If only I had tried sooner it could have been so different.

I came downstairs and found Stephen in the kitchen, preparing the evening meal. He asked, 'Why are you crying?' When I told him what the social worker had told me he replied, 'I am sure it is for the best, as I think she would have caused us so many problems. She would have been such an embarrassment.' He reminded me what Miss McFadden had said at our meeting, 'Just get on with your life.'

He appeared quite dismissive and very unsupportive, and said how he was so glad that he hadn't told his own mother or father about my adoption. Yet again my adoption was being surrounded by secrecy and shame. I felt so angry at his reaction. He didn't have any understanding of how I was actually feeling.

'Why are you still crying? At least it's an end to it now,' he said, continuing to rub salt into the wounds. 'It's not as if you actually knew her, anyway.'

Realising that I was going to have very little sympathy, I went to bed early that night. Listening to the rain falling against the window pane I eventually cried myself to sleep.

In the morning the rain had almost stopped. I still felt extremely upset by the news I had received the day before. I woke with a hollow feeling in the pit of my stomach. It was as if I was going through some kind of grieving process, but I hadn't even met the person I was mourning. It was one of the weirdest feelings I have ever had.

I got myself ready and went out, not really having any idea where I was actually going. Then I remembered that John had mentioned how he could help me find my mother's grave. I decided to drive to the cemetery nearest to where my mother had lived. I felt alone in the world, but it was something I just needed to do. I started crying for what might have been as I walked around the graveyard, not really knowing what I could possibly find.

Then I realised that she wouldn't even have had a headstone, as she had no family to buy one. Seeing the headstones with 'beloved mother' just made me cry even more. I had to stop torturing myself. What really pulled at my heart more than anything was that I would never be able to say, *Hello, Mum. I'm Phyllis, your daughter.* But I knew walking around a cemetery was not the answer. I had to accept what I had been told by John and he was right: we had reached the end of the road.

A few months went by, and I was adjusting to the fact that it was likely my birth mother had died. I was doing my best to get back to some type of normality, and I am pleased to say I didn't feel the need to make another trip to the cemetery.

I was therefore astonished when one afternoon I had a phone call from John. As usual we exchanged pleasantries, and he apologised for not having been in touch sooner. He went on to explain how heavy his workload had been, because a colleague had been off sick. I had some degree of sympathy for his hectic schedule but my curiosity was getting the better of me.

He must have recognised my slight irritation, or maybe the urgency in my voice, as he quickly changed the subject and asked if I was sitting down. He had something to tell me. I reassured him that I was prepared for whatever it was.

'Well,' he said, with a deep sigh, 'prepare yourself for a shock. Against all odds, your birth mother Bridget Ryan is still very much alive.'

I was speechless. John gave me a few moments to take in what he had just told me. I didn't know whether to laugh or cry. I told him that I had assumed my mother must have died as he'd suggested. He explained how he had decided to make one last attempt to try and see if my mother was still alive. Before he would give me her address I had to promise him that I would not try to go there on my own. Knowing how impatient I had been with the previous address in Coventry, he was not taking any chances.

My mother was living in Runcorn Road, Balsall Heath. John said that as she had changed her name to Ryan while hiding from the police, he thought she must have had a criminal record. 'Your mother is well known to the probation service in Balsall Heath and is currently on probation for causing criminal damage while being drunk and disorderly,' he told me.

It was strange hearing such a terrible thing about my own mother, and to think that only ten minutes before I had thought she was dead. It sounded like she was not just alive, she was causing mayhem! John continued to explain how he had already phoned Bridget's probation officer and had spoken to her for some time. 'She is called Bernadette, and is Irish herself. She seems to like your mother, and gets on well with her. Bridget visits her every Wednesday.'

Bernadette was only too happy to arrange a meeting and John said he thought she was eager to meet me, 'I expect she is curious to see if you resemble your mother in any way.'

I replied, 'Well I hope I'm a little better behaved than her!' I thanked him for his perseverance and told him that I would keep him informed of any further developments.

It was reassuring to hear for the first time that somebody seemed to like my mother. The whole thing was surreal and I needed a few days to absorb the information.

I was feeling apprehensive about meeting Bernadette, so when I telephoned her and she told me that she would not be able to see me for a further month, I was secretly relieved. It did feel strange talking to somebody who knew my mother so well. She was very friendly and appeared down to earth.

I kept myself busy and tried to put to the back of my mind that soon I would be meeting someone who had actually met my mother. The meeting was arranged for July 1980.

***

It was a beautiful sunny day when I met Bernadette. I was worried about the meeting, conscious that I would be under close scrutiny, but she soon put me at ease. In fact she greeted me with a hug, and I felt like her long-lost friend. Her office was small and cramped, with documents all over the desk – how she ever found anything I will never know – but she assured me that she knew where every single piece of paper was.

We enjoyed a cold drink together, which I appreciated as it was very stuffy. To make things worse she chain-smoked. She asked if I minded but I could hardly complain as she was kind enough to see me. It was obvious from the pile on her desk she had a huge workload.

We chatted for what seemed ages. She joked how I was a chatterbox like my mother, although she did most of the talking.

I asked if my mother usually sat on the same chair I was sitting on. I suppose it seemed like rather an odd question but I just felt I needed to know. She laughed but realised the importance of the meeting and the effect it was having on me. In mid-conversation she inhaled deeply on her cigarette and blew out a cloud of smoke that filled the small room. 'Yes, the very chair. We haven't got room for another one!'

There was a pause for a while as she stared at me. She apologised and said she hoped she was not making me feel uncomfortable, and then suddenly blurted out, 'I can't believe you're Bridget's daughter!'

I asked if she thought we resembled each other. She thought hard, putting her hand to her mouth while she continued to concentrate, mainly looking at my face.

'Come to think of it you do look a bit like her. You have the same cheekbones.'

For the first time in my life I actually looked like another person. It was a feeling I'd never had before. I believe she did answer my question honestly and she wasn't saying it just to make me feel better.

Bernadette told me as much as she knew about my mother, and I felt comforted by the fact that she really did seem to have a soft spot for her. She said, 'Your mother's a real character. In fact I'd even say she's a bit eccentric. She speaks very loud, almost shouting at times, and everyone in the office can usually hear her. She has a strong, distinctive, Tipperary accent, which is where she originally comes from.

'She's known as Tipperary Mary, as she was using

her middle name, Mary, to avoid the police. She doesn't stand any nonsense from anyone, but unfortunately that is what usually gets her into trouble. She comes to see me most Wednesday afternoons. She's always late and looks like she's just rolled out of bed. I'm afraid she has neglected herself and does look a lot older than she actually is. I try not to book other clients in after Bridget as she thinks she's there for the whole afternoon anyway.

'She enjoys having a chat and a cup of tea, and usually scrounges a few fags off me. She rambles a lot and sometimes it is hard to concentrate on what she's trying to tell me. Something certainly must have happened to her when she was much younger and living in Ireland, but it seems as if it is far too painful for her to talk about it.

'She goes from one subject to another and never wants to talk about why she keeps re-offending. Bridget seems to forget that is the main reason why she is meant to be visiting me!' Bernadette laughed, 'She shouts, "Off with yez, I haven't come to talk about all that now."'

Her mood changed as she said, 'It's so difficult to work with someone who is not prepared to change their ways, and Bridget certainly has no intention of doing that. Not for anybody. She breaks all the rules and somehow gets away with it, but she's a likeable person and I just wish I could do more to help her.'

I asked Bernadette if she ever talked about her children. 'Yes,' she said, 'non-stop. In fact that's what she talks about the most. It's so sad, she has so many regrets. We often carry regrets connected with our circumstances and I believe that is the main reason why Bridget turned to drink in the first place.'

Bernadette continued to explain that when Bridget had a drink she became violent and usually started fighting. 'She is often paranoid and thinks people are talking about her. She sometimes talks about Timothy, the man she lodges with. He's from Dublin and according to her he lies in bed most of the day. She says he's "a lazy idiot and a bully". It appears that Bridget has never been respected by any man in her life.'

It was a lot for me to take in. At times I almost forgot that it was actually my own mother we were talking about. Maybe it was an attempt on my part to protect myself from getting too hurt. In a strange way I was rather envious of Bernadette. She knew so much about my own mother, yet to me she was a complete stranger. But for now I was reassured by her sincerity and genuine concern for my mother's welfare.

Bernadette suggested that I could come to the probation office the following Wednesday, as Bridget would be making her usual visit. She joked, 'Don't worry, you haven't got to sit on her lap! You can stand in the reception area and you will be able see her as she comes through the door.' I thought for a few minutes, but quickly declined her offer.

I really wanted to meet her, but not in that way. It would have been more than I could cope with. All the staff would know why I was there, and the first meeting with my mother would have been so public. They'd all be looking at my reaction. It would have been so embarrassing and I wouldn't even be able to speak to her. I wouldn't be able to touch her or hug her, or say, 'Hello, I'm Phyllis your daughter.'

I thanked Bernadette for giving me so much of her time, as I knew she was running well over schedule. I told her I would give some thought to what she had suggested, but in reality I knew that was not the way I wanted to meet my mother for the first time. When I stood up, she gripped my hand and gave me a look I have never forgotten, not of pity, something deeper than that. I left the office without saying a word, but I was feeling overwhelmed by the whole experience.

***

A few weeks went by before another meeting was arranged with John. He seemed intrigued about how things had gone with Bernadette and commented on how well he thought I was coping with everything. If only he knew how I was really feeling.

He had an idea, 'We could meet Bridget in her local pub; just make it casual and pretend we are a normal couple popping into the pub for a drink. The pub is on the corner near where your mother lives. She's almost certain to be in there, and I'm sure we will be able to recognise her.' He must have driven past her house as he seemed to know the area well.

Trying to persuade me, he continued, 'A few drinks might settle your nerves and it could really turn out to be a positive meeting.' I still wasn't convinced so I told him I really needed time to think about things and I would keep in touch.

I didn't keep my word and eventually lost contact with John as there was no more he could do to help me. He knew I was determined to meet my mother one day, but I felt it was best if I did it alone, without his involvement.

***

It was now January and I was delighted to find out I was expecting my first baby in September that year. My own flesh and blood! Another human being who might even take after me. Meeting my mother would have to be postponed. I did not want to risk harming the baby or myself, as I knew meeting her would be a big shock.

I gave birth to a healthy baby boy on 9 September 1981, and we called him Stuart. I felt very emotional after the birth, realising how difficult things must have been for my own mother. To think she had gone through the whole pregnancy, the labour pains and all that entails, only one day to have to give her baby away. But I had my baby, who needed love and attention. He was amazing and I loved him instantly. He was perfect in every way.

While I was still at home with Stuart I started to think about what the first meeting with my mother might be like, and I had a recurring dream. I was pushing a baby (I assumed it was Stuart) in a big navy-blue pram, the old fashioned type with the big four wheels. When I arrived at the paper shop I always carefully put the brakes on, leaving my baby fast asleep outside, by himself. This is something I would never have done in reality.

After buying a newspaper I calmly walked out of the shop and was horrified to see that the pram was missing. As I looked up the street I noticed a lady pushing the pram, she was wearing a candlewick dressing gown. I ran frantically towards her and she stood still, just staring as if she was in a trance. Nothing was said, and I would just grab the pram from the lady and walk quickly away.

When I woke up I'd be worried for Stuart, but I would also feel the woman's pain – she looked so troubled.

When Stuart was nearly two months old I took him to the morning clinic to see my colleagues. They told me that one of my patients, Lilian, had died, and that her husband Frank was starting to turn up at the clinic and really needed someone to talk to. I decided to visit him with Stuart to cheer him up.

Frank was drinking a lot that afternoon. He seemed so lonely and vulnerable, and I could see his health was deteriorating due to the alcohol. I started to think about how my mother would be lonely and vulnerable too. It made me realise I should see her sooner rather than later.

I felt the time was right to finally meet my mother. But I had given it a great deal of thought and I was certain that I couldn't just knock on the door and say, *Hello, I'm Phyllis, your long-lost daughter*. I was married and had a baby of my own to think about, and from what I had already been told – by Bernadette as well as Miss McFadden – she was not going to fit into a normal family life.

I came up with a plan of action. I was a district nurse, and part of that role was visiting patients in their home. Seeing Frank had reminded me of the confidence I had when I was doing my job. I knew I was good at my job, and at caring for people.

I realised I could meet my mother in disguise, as her nurse. As a professional I would have a reason to enter her house, because she was used to various agencies trying to help her. She wouldn't question my visit and I would feel protected behind my nurse's uniform. I knew meeting my mother would be a lot to cope with. This way I might get to know her without her realising who I actually was.

I had the address John had given to me almost two years before and I prayed that she hadn't moved. First step, I decided, was just to drive to her house and get a feel for the area.

It was a pleasant autumn morning when I told Stephen that I was visiting a friend I hadn't seen in ages. At that time the area was known as a red light district. It was something I had never experienced before: prostitutes standing on street corners in broad daylight waiting for their punters.

Bernadette had said my mother got into trouble by fighting and stealing for money or booze, but now I wondered if she had ever been a prostitute. Was that the real reason why she had been running from the police? I stopped myself. I was determined not to judge her. I wanted to be able to help her, and not jump to the wrong conclusions before I had even had the chance to meet her. I checked my A to Z and set off.

The houses I visited as a district nurse were often in need of a lick of paint and a little scruffy, to say the least. The patients were usually old and frail, and unable to maintain their own properties as they once had. But nothing could have prepared me for the state of my mother's house.

The net curtains looked almost black, probably due to years of heavy smoking. They were only half covering the downstairs windows and I was certain that was how it had been for a very long time. The upstairs window appeared to have a dark grey blanket covering it, maybe an attempt to block out the outside world.

The house was so neglected it actually looked as if nobody could possibly be living there. I could only imagine what state the inside of the house must have been in. Did she really live in these awful conditions? Maybe the house was derelict and nobody was living there?

I felt like turning the car around and going back home to my own baby, but I knew that would be something I'd live to regret. I had come this far and I just had to see it through.

I stared at the house for about 20 minutes. My mother was probably still in bed as Bernadette had said she never got up early as she was usually hung-over from the previous night. I suddenly thought to myself, what if she comes out of the house and recognises me as her daughter? I pulled myself together. I was now a 25-year-old mother myself and the probability of her knowing me would be extremely slim.

I started to feel a little uneasy, sitting in the car by myself. I was not wearing my nurse's uniform for me to hide behind. I felt vulnerable, especially as there were prostitutes actually standing on the corner. Already a few men had passed my car and stared into the window as they passed. I felt I was drawing attention to myself and I could feel my heart racing.

I took a deep breath in an attempt to calm myself down and drove away quickly, swerving to avoid an oncoming car which I narrowly missed. To have had a collision outside my mother's house was something I definitely didn't want to happen. I realised then I would have to save all my strength for the following week and concentrate on what I had to face. The next time I was to drive down my mother's road I would be visiting as her district nurse.

I didn't tell anyone that I had driven to my mother's home. A part of me wanted to run away and never go back to that run-down derelict house. How could anyone live in such terrible conditions? I checked the address. Perhaps I had got it wrong. Had it all been a dreadful mistake? But Bridget did live in that house and there was no going back. I had come this far, and had waited a long time to meet my own flesh and blood.

Bernadette had said that Bridget was always talking about her children and was full of regrets. I hoped I would be able to give her some reassurance, and hopefully make her happier when she saw how I had turned out.

It was important that she understood I wasn't there

to judge her as a person or criticise. I knew that within my nurse's role I would be protected and I would feel less vulnerable in whatever situation I was about to find. It would be another week before I was to meet her and it seemed like an eternity.

I concentrated on looking after my own baby. It was important that I stayed in control, since this little individual was depending on me. He gave me the strength to remain focused on what was important and not to become too affected by what I was to face.

The day dawned. I had some time free before I started back at work part time, and I was finally going to meet my own mother.

All my life I had yearned to have a blood relative, another person who might have something in common with me. Now, within two months, I would have two relatives with whom I might share some inherited traits. I don't think most people can understand what it means not to have one single person in the world connected to you by blood.

It was a windy Monday morning early in November 1981, and only days away from my mother's birthday. She must have been 53 when I met her, which is younger than I am today. I got dressed in my uniform as if I was off to work as usual, but I felt as if I was role-playing, pretending to be something I wasn't.

The timing wasn't great, but I suppose there never would have been a right time. I'd just gone back to work part time after having my son, and I was feeling emotional about having to leave him with his child-minder. I also kept thinking of what my birth mother must have gone through: the labour pains, followed by the agony of having to give me up. I had bonded with Stuart so well and it was difficult to leave him, even for four hours. Yet my mother had kept me until I was eight months old before she decided to take me to the orphanage. I couldn't imagine what she must have gone through. Life must have been so hard for her.

I had thought it was best if I didn't go entirely by myself, and Stephen had agreed to accompany me to the address. I got Stuart ready and gave him his feed. He was a good baby, and usually slept for several hours, so I was keeping my fingers crossed that today would be no different. I put him in his carrycot, strapped into the car. As a baby he obviously had no idea that his mother was about to meet his grandmother for the very first time, and didn't know how she was feeling!

Stephen tried to make light conversation as he was driving us. I suppose it was his attempt to keep me occupied so that I would not dwell too much on what was about to happen. But I wasn't really listening to a word he was saying. I only had one thing on my mind – I was about to meet my mother for the very first time.

When we arrived at the house I had seen the week before I froze. My throat was dry and no words would come out of my mouth. Eventually I heard my husband say, 'I think that must be your mother's house.' He was staring at me, awaiting some kind of reaction. I felt my stomach heave. It was as if I was about to jump out of an aeroplane instead of simply stepping out of a car.

There was no turning back, and I knew I needed at least to appear as if I could deal with the situation. I straightened my uniform, checking the fob watch and pens I kept in my top pocket. Briefly touching the badge that I always wore with pride on the lapel of my blazer, I gripped my nurse's bag and diary very tightly and concentrated on detaching myself from the situation. I'd never had to visit a patient quite like Bridget before.

It may sound strange, but from my first visit I always referred to my mother as Bridget. It was a way of protecting myself from who she really was. I took a deep breath and reminded myself of the task in hand. I was visiting Bridget Mary Ryan, a new patient on my list: DOB, 11.11.1928: Chronic Alcoholic, self-neglect and with social problems.

District nurses are often faced with problems when visiting patients. You are a visitor in their home when they are at their most vulnerable, and they need to be able to put their trust in you. With the right approach we can usually give them the reassurance they need and put them at ease. You often have to remain emotionally detached to enable you to do your job in a professional way. If you allow yourself to dwell on things too much it will start to affect you and you won't perform as well. My training was going to be well and truly tested. I had waited a long time for this day.

Stephen shouted, 'Good luck.' I smiled back anxiously. I knew that it was my inner strength I needed to draw upon and that luck was not going to play a part. Conscious that my time was limited, I took a deep breath and hurried across the road to her front door.

The house looked even worse on closer inspection. As I pushed the front gate it fell from my hand and scraped along the floor. The hinge was rusty and useless. The hedge was overgrown and almost covered a dilapidated wall surrounding the small front garden. To the right there were some old rubbish bags. The spilled contents were wet and decaying and, from the smell which stung my nostrils, they must have been there for months. As I turned, I noticed some old beer and cider cans on the ground.

I looked around, feeling really nervous about ringing the doorbell. Once I had plucked up the courage to press it I was met by a deafening silence. I shouldn't have been surprised that it wasn't working I suppose as, peering more closely, it looked like it hadn't made a sound for many years.

I tried knocking hard on the front door but still there was no reply. Now I felt really sick. Had I prepared myself for nothing? Would I never be able to meet my mother? I decided to try the house next door. They were terraced houses and the neighbour's front door was at arm's length, so I only had to lean across to press the bell. Bingo. It rang immediately.

An Asian man answered the door. I smiled politely at him, though feeling even more nervous than before. I tried to appear calm as I didn't want to arouse any suspicion about the real reason I was visiting his neighbour.

From somewhere I found my voice. 'Do you know Bridget Ryan, the woman next door?' I asked. He paused for a moment, just staring at me. Then looked me up and down, clearly clocking my nurse's uniform.

'Too bloody right I do. She's a crazy mad woman, a drunken Irish woman who should be ashamed of herself. She's a dirty bitch. I don't know why they don't just lock her up for good and throw away the key.'

I tried to calm him down, which helped me get into my role as the district nurse visiting her alcoholic patient. He clearly had a lot of pent-up anger. I realised that as soon as he saw someone he considered to be an authority figure – me on this occasion – he just had to let it out. There were tears in his eyes as he continued with his rant, but I was relieved to see he seemed to be getting a little calmer. Sadly, he was just gathering strength for the next outburst.

'I mean, it's just not fair, I have a young child to think about. She's a slag and should not be living next door to families. My wife's on the verge of a nervous breakdown.'

By now I was feeling out of my depth and losing control of the situation. And I hadn't even met my mother. My anxiety must have shown, as he then changed his

172

attitude completely. He apologised for his rant, put his hand on my shoulder, and spoke in a much calmer voice. He was clearly at the end of his tether.

'I'm sorry, love, for shouting. I know it's not your fault but can you please do something to help? Please.'

I felt upset and guilty that I was powerless to help him, but also horribly aware that I was wasting valuable time. To lighten the mood, he said, 'You can take her home with you if you like, and then you will know what we have to put up with.' I had heard enough and needed to get away. If he had known the real reason for my visit I dread to think what his reaction would have been.

It had all been a terrible shock and I was close to tears. I considered my options. I was still determined to face my mother. Drunk or sober, I had to meet her. I was her nurse, not her daughter. I just had to keep telling myself that.

I thanked him for his time and he shook his head saying, 'You will need to knock on the door hard as they don't get up until the afternoon in that house. They are usually hung-over.'

Unfortunately he continued. 'The man she lives with also drinks heavily, but he is no real trouble. He stays in the house getting drunk. You only see him going out a couple of times a week, usually to the local supermarket to buy his booze. That's all you really see of him. He keeps himself to himself and minds his own business. Not like her.'

It was obvious he was desperate to give me all the details he could, and I had no choice but to listen. 'Timmy has also had enough of her. I've often heard them arguing with each other, until the early hours of the morning sometimes. It's a wonder one of them hasn't been murdered.'

That was the last thing I needed to hear. The only person who really seemed to have any time for Bridget was Bernadette, her probation officer. I glanced next door but there didn't seem to be any movement. I was surprised that they hadn't heard the neighbour shouting. I think a brass band could have been playing in the street and still they would have remained dead to the world. I suppose it was like the middle of the night for them, even though by now it was about 11 a.m. Waking two drunks before they were ready wasn't going to be an easy task.

'It's about time she got disturbed. It's like waking the dead in that bleeding place,' the neighbour said. Suddenly he put his hand to his mouth and gasped, as a thought struck him. 'Oh, I hope he hasn't murdered her in there. Come to think of it, I did hear a lot of shouting last night.'

Thank goodness, he then went inside. I turned once more to the shabby navy blue front door and peered through the letterbox. I could see straight into the front room as there was no hallway. In the corner was an unmade bed, topped by an old stained mattress and a torn, discoloured sheet that had seen much better days.

Could that be my mother's bed, where she lay in the early hours in a drunken stupor? There was a pile of old newspapers stacked in one corner, and the bit of carpet you could see was filthy and threadbare. It was in a terrible state, and the smell took my breath away.

I continued rattling the rusty old letterbox and nearly jumped out of my skin when I heard a shout from the back room.

'The fecking door's open, ya eejit, how many times do you need to be told?'

I wasn't exactly expecting them to get the red carpet out but I was shocked by the rudeness of the man I assumed to be Timmy. At this point I really did feel like running away. He must have opened the door when I was talking to the neighbour. I pushed hard and for the first time in my life, walked into my mother's home.

The feeling I had on that memorable day in November 1981 was one I will never forget. It was a mixture of terror, anticipation and excitement. I was now only minutes away from meeting my mother for the very first time and there was no going back.

I tried to introduce myself to Timmy but I was stammering and my heart was thumping following his outburst. I needed to stay calm. It was crucial that I didn't expose my true identity. Timmy was not a man for formalities, so I was aware of the importance of acting in a professional manner while maintaining my role as Bridget's district nurse.

It worked. My visit wasn't even questioned. He wasn't at all bothered about why I'd come, but I had rehearsed my lines for weeks and was determined at least to have the chance to explain the reason for my visit. He didn't bat an eyelid when I said, 'I've come to visit Bridget Ryan to see how she is.'

Timmy was standing in the small kitchen. This led through to the middle room, which had hardly any furniture apart from a clapped-out armchair. There were no pictures or ornaments to make it feel a bit more homely. An old gas fire fixed in the fireplace had been turned up to its highest setting, and the heat from it was quite overpowering. At least they were able to keep warm, and weren't worried about their fuel bills.

In the corner was the door leading to the stairs. Timmy sat down on what I supposed was his armchair and lit a cigarette. He inhaled deeply and let the ash fall to the floor where his scuffed trainers rubbed it into the threadbare carpet. It was obvious he was a heavy smoker by the rattle in his chest and the yellow nicotine stains on his fingers. There he sat, this scruffy old man in a dirty grey singlet covering his enormous beer belly, and shabby brown trousers coming apart at the seams.

'She's a damned nuisance and a disgrace to the Irish population,' he bellowed. I wondered whether he had looked in the mirror at himself lately.

Trying to hurry things along, I asked, 'Is the lady upstairs?', which got him going again.

'O God, she's certainly no lady and never has been.'

It was on the tip of my tongue to say, *well you're certainly no gentleman*! But I didn't want to antagonise him.

Eventually Timmy shouted from the bottom of the stairs, 'There's a young lady to see you.' Turning to check, and looking a little puzzled for the first time as to who I actually was, he continued, 'I think she's a nurse.'

I could hear a lot of banging from upstairs and I wasn't sure whether a large, heavy object had fallen. There was certainly a lot of noise coming from the bedroom where my mother presumably was. I waited patiently, trying to appear calm but my heart was pounding even harder and I was sweating profusely.

As Bridget walked down the stairs, or rather banged down each step, with every thud I heard I knew that she was that bit closer to me. The moment I had anticipated for so long was now only seconds away. I couldn't wait another minute, so I peered around the corner, trying to see if I could at least get a glimpse of her.

The light was poor and the stairs were steep, but I spotted her sitting on a step, as if exhausted. I stood back, and suddenly the door flung open with some considerable force and there she stood. My own mother was standing there in front of me.

It was as if she was someone else. Even though I had been told what to expect, for some reason I just couldn't, or wouldn't, believe that this poor crumpled creature was indeed my mother.

'Are you Bridget?' I asked. Half of her face was swollen and badly bruised, and her left eye was black, perhaps from a recent fight or a fall. Her hair was grey and smelled of stale alcohol and tobacco. It was thickly matted at the back, as if it hadn't been washed or combed for months. She was wearing a semi-transparent short nylon nightdress in what had once been a luminous colour, revealing mottled rings on her legs caused by sitting too close to the fire. Her finger nails were filthy as if she had been digging up potatoes and I could see she was also a heavy smoker as she had yellow nicotine stains on her fingers.

I stood staring at her for a short time, almost in disbelief. Years of abusing her body had clearly taken its toll. I felt sorry for her. It was clear that alcohol was now completely controlling her life and that she had lost all self-respect and self-control. I peered at her face, looking for some similarity, some sign of myself in this human wreck. Yes, I thought, there is some likeness there – the cheekbones perhaps, the tilt of the chin. This was my mother, and I was determined to recognise her.

I felt very emotional, but I pulled myself up sharply. I needed to remind myself that this was Bridget Ryan, my patient, not my mother. Thankfully Bridget didn't even seem to notice.

By this time Timmy decided to go back into the front room where he actually slept on that dirty old mattress. He grunted something under his breath, which I'm sure was to do with Bridget irritating him.

He complained that he was feeling very tired and 'was never allowed to get any sleep in this damn place'. That didn't surprise me, as I'm sure he had used what little energy he had in complaining about Bridget and how he couldn't possibly live with her for a minute longer.

Bridget still had her strong Tipperary accent, despite having lived in England for over 28 years. She was delighted to have a nurse visit her. She needed people to talk to: people who were prepared to listen. She led me into a room with clothes all over the floor and dirty plates left from the previous day. There was rubbish piled in carrier bags, and the curtains were still firmly drawn.

As she launched into her life story, I hardly said a word, not a word. I just stared. She really liked to talk; maybe she did that all the time to anyone who was prepared to listen. I certainly was a good listener for her that day.

I wonder if it was some kind of strange telepathy because, within moments of our meeting, Bridget began talking about a girl she had given away once, called Phyllis.

'Ah, she was a lovely baby, a lovely child. I miss her, even now I miss her.' She told me about other children, but didn't want to dwell on them and it all seemed rather muddled.

The one she kept coming back to was me. I thought maybe it was because she had looked after me for eight months and perhaps the others had been taken away from her much sooner. She rambled on about how much she wanted to find Phyllis again; how the orphanage had refused to tell her where her daughter was. She even told me about the letter she had written in 1973. She remembered the name of the orphanage and she remembered my birthday, which meant so much to me.

She didn't ask me any questions, not even why I had come to visit her. I expect she was just so glad to have someone to talk to – a sympathetic listener. She didn't even ask my Christian name – I realised I hadn't prepared myself with an alternative, so that was lucky.

Strangely enough, I don't remember the very first words she said to me, but I do remember how talkative she was. Her Irish accent fascinated me, but at times I found it difficult to understand. She talked so fast and was jumping from one subject to another within seconds. She seemed happy to have a visitor, which made me feel sad. It was obvious that she was very lonely.

Bernadette had told me a lot about Bridget and seemed to know more about her than anyone, so at least I had been able to prepare myself. She had warned me that she rambled, and it could sometimes be difficult to understand what she was trying to say. I now knew what she meant.

Bridget was certainly very loud, and she suddenly shouted at me. 'What are you staring at me for?' This really unsettled me. It was obvious that she often drew attention to herself by the way she looked, and her booming voice was something that you could never ignore. This had caused her to become paranoid, and she always believed that people were staring at her, judging her by the way she looked and spoke.

I was actually thinking that I had seen her somewhere before, but I felt confused and overwhelmed. I dismissed the thought as I felt it was just going to make things more complicated.

It was some years later when I realised that my

mother had actually been that drunken Irish woman from Tipperary who had been brought into A & E in 1975 after being involved in a fight.

Now, I quickly smiled and leant across to stroke her arm. A part of me longed to say, 'I'm here. I am Phyllis, your missing daughter.' I could only imagine the joy I would have given my mother. But a more sensible voice kept warning me that this was not the time. Maybe there would never be a right time, but it certainly wasn't then.

She soon calmed down and continued to tell her story, interspersed with muddled and bizarre asides. She turned suddenly to me and began asking questions. Was I married? Did I have any children? Oh, if only she knew, I thought to myself, and several times I could hardly resist telling her. It seemed so cruel not to, yet I knew I had to restrain myself. My husband and son were waiting outside in the car.

I so wanted to stay longer but I had said that the first visit would be quite short, and I was aware that I must have been running well over my time. I promised I would call again soon, hopefully in two weeks' time. Bridget smiled and said how much she liked me and she would look forward to seeing me again.

I would love to have kissed her but it might have seemed odd. As I was leaving, she stroked my hair and attempted to remove it from my eyes, the type of thing a mother might do. She seemed affectionate towards me. Maybe it was because I took the time to listen to her, but we somehow seemed to make a connection.

Coming away from the house I thought about her, I had liked her at once. She really seemed glad to be able to have someone to talk to. If only she had realised that it was her own daughter. I was glad that I seemed to be so important to her, even after all this time. For better or worse, at last I had finally met my mother.

Chapter 8

Caring for My Mother

I had now met my birth mother, and needed some time to reflect on what I'd found.

Had I introduced myself as her long-lost daughter I'm sure she would have thrown her arms around me. I knew she wasn't a sensible, rational person. I could easily imagine her turning up on my doorstep day and night – highly intoxicated and singing at the top of her voice – the way she did outside her own house. Once that door was open I knew I'd never get her out of my life. More than that, if I had to try I knew it would hurt her too much. I could already tell she'd be so glad to have found one of her children.

On the other side of the coin, I really didn't want to turn my back on her just because she wasn't the mother I had been hoping for. I had liked her instantly. I wanted her to be able to confide in me as she seemed tortured by the events of the past, and was full of regrets about all her children. I suppose I saw myself as her advocate. I was the one person who cared enough about her and wanted to try and help as much as possible.

The fact that I was a nurse and had experience of dealing with people like her was a distinct advantage. People are often frightened by alcoholics or down-and-outs when they act strangely. They can have differing degrees of mental health problems, but I had always warmed to their vulnerability. I've never been afraid, and find their innocence touching. They are often unable to make decisions for themselves, and need help. I was glad I had found my mother. I decided I would continue to visit her as her 'district nurse', and hoped I would be able to give her the help she desperately needed.

But first we needed to get to know each other, and hopefully in time she would learn to trust me. I wanted to be her nurse, her friend, and maybe even one day her daughter. I never regretted tracing her, even for a moment.

I knew I should visit Bridget again soon; there needed to be some continuity of my role as her district nurse.

I picked a Friday afternoon about ten days later – I thought that at least she should be out of bed at that time of day.

What I hadn't prepared myself for was, again, the next door neighbour. I parked my car a few doors away, and as I started walking to Bridget's front door I saw him standing outside his house with his arms folded, looking extremely annoyed. He was determined that I was going to listen to what he had to say.

He invited me in by unfolding his arms and placing his hand on my shoulder, so as to divert me to his own front door. I told him I was in a rush and had a lot of other patients to visit, but he reassured me that he wouldn't keep me long and insisted that I went into his house. He introduced himself as Neil and offered me a cup of tea. I declined, since I was on my lunch break from work and really didn't have much time. I sat down on a chair in his front room, fearing that if I didn't I might collapse as I was so worried about the situation I had got myself into.

I was there under false pretences and realised my true identity might be exposed. I was also terrified of what he was about to tell me about my mother. Thankfully, he didn't ask me any questions, not even my name or where I was from; he seemed more intent on telling me about the problems he had living next door to this 'horrible Irish drunken woman'.

He appeared extremely anxious. Once again he told me how awful his life was living next door to such a 'bitch', and he became more verbally aggressive. I had no choice but to listen to what he wanted to tell me as he had so much pent-up anger inside him which he needed to release.

'This should never be allowed to happen,' he said. 'A mad woman living amongst normal people, I mean, would you want to live next door to such a horrible person?' He gave me no chance to reply before the next stream of words poured out.

He talked about her singing and shouting in the street again. 'Many of the neighbours often open their bedroom windows and start shouting and swearing at her. She never seems to care. In fact she just starts shouting even louder and swearing back at them. She is totally unreasonable. Usually she ends up lying in the gutter, crying loudly, having no consideration or respect for anyone, least of all for herself.'

Then he spoke in a much quieter tone, even for a few moments appearing slightly sympathetic. 'I think something really bad must have happened to her, and that is why she turned to drink.'

There was so much he wanted to tell me but I really didn't want to hear such terrible things about my own mother. I got up from the chair, but he didn't even notice and just continued, almost in a whisper, as if he thought she could hear what he was telling me through the walls.

'I think all her children were put into care years ago. The woman a few doors away, she has not long had a baby girl. Well, her husband was so angry a few weeks ago that he shouted at her – Bridget – to shut up, telling her she was a selfish woman who was going to wake up their baby.

'We just couldn't believe her reaction. She was really drunk as usual and shouting at the top of her voice. Then she started screaming and was crying hysterically that she had babies once, but they were all taken away from her.'

He told me how she'd fallen to the ground and was sobbing uncontrollably, screeching as loudly as she could, 'Why did they take my babies away?' She was lying in the alley. He even walked to the window and moved the net curtain to show me the exact spot. I couldn't bear to look at where my own mother had lain in a drunken stupor, crying for her lost children. It was more than I could have coped with, as by now I was feeling sick and wanted to run out of the house. I just couldn't bear to hear any more, and I knew he must never find out that I was indeed one of those children that had been put into care.

But still he was determined to tell me more. 'One of the neighbours must have called the police. We went out to check if she was OK as she suddenly went quiet and seemed lifeless. Nobody wanted to touch her or get involved as she was so dirty. She smelt, had vomit all over her, and was often quite violent. She would kick out if you as much as stood next to her. She was crazy and acted like a wild animal. By the time the police arrived she was ranting and raving and then started swearing at them to "fecking leave me alone".'

Neil apologised for the language, then said, 'I don't know why they didn't just leave her to choke on her own vomit.' It was obvious he hated what she was and desperately wanted her out of the area, but it was difficult for me to have to listen to him. I had some degree of sympathy with what he was going through. I didn't want her turning up at my door disturbing my baby boy, after all, but I wasn't the right person to give him the help he needed, and I was petrified that he might find out my true identity.

But there was no stopping him. 'The police arrested her for being drunk and disorderly although that's an understatement to say the least. She is an utter disgrace to the human race and thank God her kids were put into care,' he said. If only he knew, I thought to myself.

Still he turned the knife. 'When she was eventually carted off in a police van everybody was cheering and clapping. It was better than any episode of Coronation Street.' He then started sniggering as if he was telling me a joke, but I certainly wasn't amused. I mustered some degree of confidence and professionalism, saying, 'I really need to leave now.'

As I started to walk away, he said, 'All the neighbours were so pleased, me included, as we thought she had been taken away for good – but no such luck. Within a few days she was back, making a bloody nuisance of herself again.'

I just wanted to get out of his house as quickly as possible. Even if I still had time, I wasn't in any fit state to visit Bridget that day. Neil did eventually apologise for keeping me so long, but even as I walked out of the front door he was still making one last desperate attempt to make me listen. 'Please see what you can do to help me get rid of this awful woman,' he said. I hurriedly returned to my car, desperate to get away from such a complicated situation.

The next week, I really hoped that Neil wouldn't be standing at the gate. I was also crossing my fingers that my mother would be at home. Thankfully he was nowhere to be seen, and my mother was actually in. Remembering how difficult it was to rouse them on my previous visit, I knocked the door hard. After a few minutes, Timmy in his by now familiar, disgruntled voice was shouting, 'Will ya fecking wait a minute, for God's sake!'

I'd already established that he wasn't one for formalities. Again he appeared irritated by my visit, but I reminded myself that I'd come to visit Bridget, not him, and I ignored his rudeness. He stared at me in the same way as before, then acknowledged my nurse's uniform. Timmy, grunting something along the lines of 'she's in the back kitchen,' promptly lay back on his horrible grubby bed.

The house had a musty smell; a combination of dust

and alcohol, and still looked like a bombsite. I prepared myself to meet my mother for the second time professionally. I still needed to remain detached from the circumstances, but I already loved her as my mother. I realised she was often difficult, that she would fly off the handle for no reason and was also very highly strung and impulsive. But she was so pathetic that you could almost excuse her bad behaviour. Once again, I tried to remind myself, it was Bridget, a patient I had come to see; not my mother.

I went through to the back kitchen where she stood against the dilapidated work surface, next to a very greasy, dirty gas cooker. She bent her head over the naked flame to light her cigarette, almost setting her hair alight in the process. Her fingers were copper-brown from years of heavy smoking, and her lipstick was smeared around her mouth. Her hair remained tangled but the swelling and bruising on her face had disappeared. For a moment I was shocked, as I could now distinguish her pale, emaciated face as she looked up at me. She was exhausted and weary after years of abusing her body.

I didn't say a word. I just sat down carefully on a battered chair that had one leg missing. Looking around, I could see filth and rubbish everywhere, so I got up and helped to tidy the place a little, but was careful not to appear as if I was interfering. Then I sat back down and listened again to her life story.

This time I managed to ask a few questions, but was careful not to arouse suspicion by seeming too nosey. Bridget was delighted to have such a keen, sympathetic listener.

'Who was Phyllis's father?' I asked with some trepidation, but Bridget seemed happy to tell me. She had met him in an Irish night club in Hurst Street, Birmingham. He was lovely, she said. She'd been going out with him for three weeks when he suggested a weekend away in a hotel.

She said she took a real fancy to him; he was a 'real attractive man'. She didn't go with men usually, not in those days, but he was special, and she loved him, she said. She hoped he would stay and that she'd keep him but, after the weekend, he disappeared – he didn't want to see her again. According to my mother, that was how I was conceived. After she gave me away, her life changed. After that it was, she said, 'more or less any old man, and she didn't mind who', but Phyllis's father, well he'd been something special. She kept saying that.

Maybe that is why she talked about Phyllis the most.

I remembered what she had told the orphanage, and although this version was slightly different, where she had met my father remained the same.

The description of events that she gave me seemed sincere and I'd like to believe that she had at least one loving encounter during her lifetime. Maybe I was conceived out of love after all, at least as far as Bridget was concerned. I'm sure that she had deliberately decided not to give the nuns all the details about my father, since it may well have just complicated things, especially if he was a married man, which she suspected was the case.

Suddenly Bridget stared in my direction and gave me a half-hearted smile. She looked straight into my face and asked, 'What's your name?' I told her I was called Pat, which was the first name that came into my head. It was a strange feeling having to pretend that I had a different name. I suppose it really rubbed it in that I had to see myself in the third person. However, she instantly forgot my name was 'Pat' and from that day on she always referred to me as her nurse, which made things easier.

After Christmas I started to visit her once or twice a month. It would be mostly in the afternoons, as I knew she'd be awake and I'd have finished work for the day. I always felt a bit guilty that I was leaving my son with the childminder for an extra hour.

I'd bring a sandwich from the supermarket sometimes, but she'd just say 'leave it there' and I never knew if she'd eat it. I tried to take some clothes, but I had to be careful not to offend her. Sometimes she'd be out, and I'd have got all worked up to see her and then have to hurry away to avoid Neil.

When she was in I gave her support, but I was really just someone to talk to. It was lovely that there was banter between us, but sometimes she needed medical attention. She quite often had burns on her legs from the fire, so I'd tend to them, and her cuts and bruises from drinking, although she wasn't keen on me making a fuss.

Once I brought a bowl through so I could try to clean and cut her fingernails. She flung it out of my hand and said, 'Take that fecking bowl out.'

I said, 'I just thought I'd give you a manicure.' She looked at me like I was mad!

She'd ignore me when I tried to give her advice. 'Why have you taken your dressings off?' I'd ask her, and she'd blame Timmy or say, 'They're better now aren't they?'

Timmy would ask, sounding jealous, 'Why does she need a dressing?' Although sometimes he'd just be snoring his head off.

When she was very drunk, it was difficult to be around her. I'd go if it was clear I'd outstayed my welcome. Every time I'd think I was two steps into helping her, building the relationship, she'd knock me right back.

Often I wanted to put my arm around her and tell her the truth. But I had a young baby and was married, we wanted another baby.

Normally I would be playing two parts. When I was at home I was Mum and Phyllis. At work I was the district nurse. With Bridget it was something else again, and I couldn't tell anybody. I had no one to confide in.

One day I asked her why she never wanted to go back to Ireland. She fixed me with one of her stares for a few minutes without saying a word, and I regretted asking her the question. Her face was tormented, and she started whispering as if she was worried that Timmy might overhear. 'My brother's a wicked man. He threatened to kill me once, if ever I told anyone.' Now I felt scared. What could be so bad that he'd threatened her in that way?

It was difficult for me to follow what she was saying then, as she kept losing her thread and peppering her comments with bizarre asides. 'They're after me all the time. For sex. They all want me. I often have one night stands. Any man will do. Drinking makes it easy. It doesn't matter if they are married or single, but they are usually Irish. Even the Asian men seem to be after me now.'

I did not want to hear this from my own mother. What can her brother have done to her to make her this way? Why did she allow herself to be used by so many men? Was it because she was always in a haze of booze, or did she use the drink to drown it all out? Love just never came into it. I always knew that something led to her alcoholism and she drank largely to blot out whatever was gnawing at her. Saying I'd be back to visit her within the next two weeks, I let myself out, with the sound of Timmy snoring in the background as I shut the front door behind me.

I continued to visit her regularly, and as the months went on I often took her new clothes, towels, sheets and food. She had long gone beyond pride about accepting charity and was always pleased when I took her new outfits which she needed badly.

Timmy remained surly, and less than pleased with my visits. He grumbled that I gave him no warning, no time to clean up the place. He was ashamed to have it seen like this. I couldn't imagine him ever cleaning up, however much notice I gave, but I tried to make him feel that I was not criticising the way he and my mother lived. I often cleaned and tidied a little but, I hoped, not in a way that he would regard as a rebuke or act of disapproval.

It was autumn 1983, and when I called, Timmy told me that Bridget was back in prison again, for shoplifting. I thought to myself, at least she won't be drinking, and will have a hot meal inside her.

For once Timmy seemed glad to see me. He said his back ached badly, so I saw to him and listened to his grumbles. I took the opportunity to ask him a little more about my mother, but once I thought I saw him looking at me oddly. For a moment I feared he had recognised the resemblance and any minute he would accuse me of being who I really was, her own child. I was convinced that I looked so much like my mother that anyone could spot it.

But he didn't. He told me, 'She used to help around the house, doing the washing and the shopping. Bridget was useful at first when I agreed to take her in. She even sometimes cooked meals, but things have gone from bad to worse. She was only meant to stay for a short time, but now I can't get rid of her. She's been barred from all the local pubs because of her aggressive behaviour. She threatens the other customers and intimidates them. At least when she did go to the pub I'd have a few hours' peace without her bothering me.'

By now he was really feeling sorry for himself. 'She's well known at the local supermarket as "Tipperary Mary", one of the Irish alkies from up the road.' He appeared baffled by who else they may have been talking about – who these other 'Irish alkies' were, which made me smile as he was Irish and spent most of his waking hours drinking. He always seemed to see himself as superior to Bridget.

I had sometimes seen Bridget walking along the road with her tartan shopping trolley on wheels, full of cans of lager and cider, which she'd just picked up from the supermarket. I never saw any sign of food in her trolley, just alcohol. Timmy told me it was now causing problems as the regular customers didn't like being in the shop with her. She was often unsteady, her words were slurred and she would shout obscenities at them. 'No one wants anything more to do with her.'

I'd heard enough for one day. My mother was in prison and a disruptive alcoholic. I retrieved my coat, resisted brushing it down and headed for the front door, raising my hand to say goodbye. 'I will come and see Bridget when she's out of prison,' I called, almost as an afterthought. For the first time he threw me a quizzical smile and almost appeared sad that I was leaving.

Timmy had said that Bridget had been sentenced to six weeks in prison, so I didn't visit for another eight weeks. It was almost two years since I'd first visited her as a district nurse, yet she still had no idea that I was her daughter. This was to be the most upsetting visit yet.

As I approached the house, Timmy had already opened the door, stepping to one side to encourage me to enter. He was shouting, 'That bloody bitch. That dirty cat! She messed herself again. I've had enough. Enough of her and her filth!'

But he was glad to see me. I went upstairs and found her lying on the bed in her own faeces, drunk, disgusting and wild. Her flesh was bruised and sore from falling over; her hair dishevelled. It was fortunate that I was a nurse, already well used to scenes of this kind. How else would I have coped?

I ran a bath with warm water, and somehow managed to help her in. While I was washing her, I noticed brown marks running down her legs, probably more diarrhoea. I gently sponged her skin until she was clean. I helped her put her right leg over the side of the bath, and she edged it gingerly on to the floor. Then the other leg.

Bridget stood motionless, dripping, her upper lip trembling with the cold as there was no heating in the bathroom. I wrapped an old grey towel around her shivering body, desperate to show her some kindness.

By pushing and pulling her I managed to guide her from the bathroom to her bedroom, where she fell back on to the stripped bed, naked, rolling over, sprawling, hideously out of control. It was the first time I had seen her in such a state of undress. I preserved her dignity by helping her to put on some reasonably clean clothes, tidied her up as best I could.

I couldn't have just left her in such a state. Again, she had scorched her legs from sitting too close to the fire, so I treated the burns and applied dressings to prevent them from becoming infected, and then we went down to the kitchen.

She began to ramble as she so often did, mainly

about sex. She repeated what she'd said so many times – all the men down the road were after her, sex mad, couldn't get enough of her, and so on.

Timmy suddenly came into the room really angry, and kept saying he'd had enough. He wanted to move out of the house and to escape from her.

'Don't you know of a home to put her in?' he kept asking me.

I became afraid now that, if he went to the authorities, he would discover that I wasn't visiting the house officially at all. I would be in deep trouble. Worse, they might guess why I had been visiting her and who I was. If he knew who I was, he would dump her on me without a moment's hesitation. It would be a matter of: 'You're her daughter, she's your responsibility, you take her in. You've got a nice house; it's your duty.'

Perhaps I could have managed her if I was on my own, but I was married and had a child to think of. As much as I wanted to in one way, I couldn't do that to them. I couldn't bring her into our lives without causing chaos, and that wouldn't be fair. She was a law unto herself. I knew that really she needed to go into a nursing home where she would be looked after, but I also knew she'd never accept that. She was only in her fifties, and functional when not drunk. If I knew that she was safely in a home then I could tell her who I really was. I desperately wanted to tell her before she died, because I knew it would make her happy.

By now, I knew she was fond of me, and I'm sure she'd have been thrilled if she knew I was Phyllis. I wanted her to know that she did the right thing leaving me at the orphanage when I was eight months old. I could reassure her that, even if it had been painful at the time, it had been the right thing for me, and that might have made her feel better about it. I wouldn't tell her that my adoptive family life hadn't been the best experience, or that I wasn't close to my adoptive mother. I didn't need to say that. I knew that clearly I had been much better off with them than I would have been with her.

I called to see Bridget the following week to make sure that she was OK. Unsurprisingly, she'd removed the dressings from her legs. She never complied with anything I asked her to do – she was the definition of a difficult patient! But I was surprised to find that the burns to her legs had healed well. Luckily they'd only been superficial.

However, the previous visit had had a huge impact. I was now eight weeks pregnant, and I had realised that

I was neither emotionally nor physically able to cope with my mother's unpredictable behaviour. I had to stay away and focus on Stuart and my pregnancy. I knew I wouldn't be visiting her for some time.

My daughter Hannah was born on 17 July 1984. Life was extremely hectic, working full time, looking after two small children, and suffering from the repercussions of meeting my mother had all taken their toll.

Perhaps I had post-natal depression. I'd have the odd glass of Christmas sherry from the cupboard in the afternoon. And a couple of times – when the children had gone to bed and Stephen was at work – I had quite a few glasses.

The reasons for my behaviour are difficult to explain. I felt confused and worried about my mother's welfare, but there was little I could do to help her.

To make matters worse, I rarely saw my adoptive mother. We just weren't close. Carole's children were a similar age to mine, so of course Carole's got more attention. I don't think my children noticed, but I did. Stephen's parents were brilliant grandparents, but they didn't know about my adoption.

Inevitably my confusion started affecting my marriage. We didn't have many friends and Stephen was often working nights. We just didn't talk to each other, the romance had gone.

On one occasion when I'd had a row with Stephen, it was about ten o'clock at night and the children were fast asleep in bed. I was angry and upset, and wanted to get away from the hostile atmosphere so I went for a drive in the car, not having any idea where I was going.

I found myself outside Bridget's house. I parked the car a few doors away and sobbed uncontrollably in the middle of the night. Although affected by the disagreement with my husband, I was even more upset that I had a mother who didn't even know I was her daughter. A mother I would never be able to talk to about my problems, as she had far too many of her own.

This was the reality check I needed. I thought to myself, For god's sake, this is nonsense. I'm not acting like a mother. *I'm acting more like my mother.* I knew I needed to bring myself to my senses. I wasn't going to change my mother's way of life, and this isn't what I wanted for my own children. I realised there was a thin dividing line between it all going horribly wrong and putting my life back in order.

I decided I could only give Bridget so much of me.

The most important thing was my two little children. Meeting my mother mustn't affect their childhood. I made the decision to stay away from her for a while to concentrate on being a mother myself. I had to put her to the back of my mind.

I stayed away from Bridget for over a year. But even though she was far removed from the longed-for mother I had hoped to find, the little girl in me still had this aching need to be with my birth mother. I felt extremely anxious about how she was continuing to cope at home.

By November 1985 I had got over the post-natal depression and was starting to see things a bit clearer. I was getting on better with Stephen, too. I felt in control again, emotionally stronger, and decided I wanted to see my mother on my terms. I really hoped that she hadn't forgotten me, the nurse who had cared for her.

As I knocked hard on the front door, which was still in the same state of disrepair, I thought back to my previous visits and how difficult it was to make them hear. This time it was obvious that there was nobody in the house, not even Timmy shouting in his usual stroppy manner. Maybe it was one of the days when he visited the local supermarket to buy his groceries, cigarettes and cans of beer.

I sat in the car for a while, checking my diary, seeing how many other patients I needed to visit that afternoon, and I tried to keep myself distracted and to stay calm. As always when visiting my mother I had to prepare myself emotionally, so that if she wasn't in I wouldn't be disappointed.

I was shocked to hear a lot of shouting. There seemed to be a brawl in the street behind where I'd parked. I quickly decided it would be better if I didn't get involved – it certainly wasn't the type of area you wanted to hang around for any length of time, especially as a woman on your own – and I tried to drive away.

As I pulled out, I looked in my rear mirror and the awful realisation hit me. It was my mother doing all the shouting. She was screeching as loudly as she could in her distinctive Tipperary accent. Timmy had told me she'd accost people in the street for no reason, and pick fights with complete strangers. She often carried an old red handbag that looked as if it had very little in it, but she would use it to hit people who so much as glanced in her direction.

On this particular afternoon it was someone who just

happened to be walking past and was probably trying their best not to make any eye contact with her, but she had assumed that they were making fun of her. Suddenly Bridget started banging the car window, shouting, 'Where are you going?' It was a strange feeling, as if she'd recognised me. I was shocked, because I hadn't seen her for a long time, although I was wearing my nurse's uniform. Maybe she was like that with everyone she met? Perhaps she normally went up to complete strangers and asked them for a lift?

I'd like to think that she did actually recognise me. It made me feel closer to her. She was so vulnerable and in a strange way I felt more attached to her because of it. I opened the car window and in her usual bossy, abrupt way she shouted at the top of her voice, 'Come on with yez, give me a lift into town.'

'Would you like me to wait for you to get ready?' I asked, trying to be subtle, but she just looked bewildered.

'Auk, what's the matter with yez? I'm as ready as I'll ever be. Just give us a lift into town, for God sake, and hurry up as I'm late as it is!'

I'm not actually sure what she was going to be late for, but I'm sure that alcohol would have been playing some part. She was often abrupt in her manner, even insulting, but in a strange way I never felt offended by her insults. It made me feel as if we were able to be ourselves around each other, just like any other mother and daughter.

I suppose I tolerated her more because of who she was to me. I accepted her behaviour better than other people. She never tried to make a good impression; the complete opposite of my adoptive mother, who spent all her life worrying about what other people might think. My birth mother had gone beyond caring whether people liked her or not. She didn't give a damn. Bridget would act the same with whoever she met.

Her behaviour was the effect of years of alcohol abuse. She'd lost all her inhibitions and was never embarrassed by her own, often inappropriate, behaviour. Most people would walk on the other side of the street just to avoid any confrontation with her. She was often stared at as if she was some kind of freak, but she had long since lost any concept of right or wrong. I was saddened by her hopelessness.

So, that afternoon I gave her a lift into town. She was so excited; it was as if we were going out for the day. I don't expect she'd been in a car for a long time. I also felt excited, if only for a very short time; it just seemed so natural.

To think I was actually giving my own mother a lift! At this point I was so close to telling her who I really was. In my head I was saying, *Come on then, Mum. Let's take you back to my house for a cup of tea and an iced bun, and you can see your grandchildren.*

I quickly came back to reality as I caught the odour from her clothes. She smelt as though she'd been sleeping rough for days and hadn't had her clothes washed in weeks. Her hands and face were filthy.

It was such a difficult time for me, but I knew I had to be strong for the sake of my own children. They needed me and no matter what, they were my main responsibility. I couldn't allow myself to become involved again, especially with her dysfunctional life. I tried to tell myself that I was just giving one of the patients a lift to the hospital for an outpatient appointment.

We soon arrived in the city centre, as it was only a short journey. I asked her if she had any money to get back home, knowing what her reply would be. She started patting her empty pockets to emphasise how broke she was. 'I've got no money, not a penny,' she said.

I gave her five pounds, knowing that it would probably be spent on alcohol and not on her journey home. I didn't want to give her any more money as when she was drunk she could so easily be mugged by the sort of people she hung around with.

As she clambered out of the car I noticed a small wet patch on the back of what had probably once been cream trousers. I thought I could smell urine, but I was trying my best not to inhale too deeply as the smell was horrible.

I noticed some teenage boys sitting on a wall, close to where I had dropped her off. They kept staring at her, and then started laughing and pointing at her. They were teasing her and calling her names. I was desperately trying not to listen to what they were shouting, but a group of teenage boys was not going to bother Bridget in the slightest. I watched her swearing and shouting back at them, swinging her handbag in their direction.

She was obviously no threat to them, and they ran in the opposite direction. A couple of them ran back towards my car and made gestures to me, as if to imply that she was a mad woman.

Maybe they thought I was her nurse and not making a very good job of looking after her. I felt really angry because of how they were mocking her; it seemed so cruel. I wanted to shout at them, *Leave her alone, that's my mother you're laughing at!* But how could I? It was upsetting and I felt guilty. I wanted to protect her. Why had I left her at the roadside to be mocked in this way?

Perhaps it hadn't been a good idea to give her a lift into town. I suppose I was just trying to do something normal with her, but maybe she would never have been the type of mother to do anything like go into town with you. It was around four years since I had found her, and it was all getting horribly out of control. Would I ever be able to tell her who I really was? I needed more time to think about things, but unfortunately that luxury was something I didn't have. My mother's mental state was deteriorating rapidly. If I was ever going to tell her who I really was, I knew it had to be soon.

When I started visiting again, some days she greeted me like a long lost friend and sometimes she'd tell me to bugger off. Her life seemed to be getting increasingly chaotic.

I didn't tell Stephen much about the meetings, and he didn't want to know. It was like she was my secret. I'd always felt protected when I made the decision to care for my mother anonymously as her nurse. I knew I could hide behind that role, wearing my uniform.

When I dropped in, Timmy was often cooking his breakfast. One day, he put it down while he went to make his tea and she grabbed it, sat down and started to eat.

He went absolutely ballistic. 'This is what I have to put up with! She's so selfish and she only thinks of herself.'

'Would you like me to cook you one, then?' I asked.

'No,' he grunted, 'I'm not hungry now.'

'Oh well, Bridget looks like she could do with a meal more than you,' I replied, looking from his beer belly to her skin and bones.

'You keep out of it,' said Timmy.

They often acted like an old married couple, and I was the child trying to keep the peace. It sometimes felt there was a special bond between the three of us.

I decided to visit my mother one afternoon when I had a little more time. It was a Monday, and Stephen was looking after Stuart and Hannah, so when I finished my official visits I called Stephen to say that work had asked me to stay on for a few hours as we had a very poorly patient.

I loved my mother now, and hoped she'd be in so I could spend more time with her. Fortunately, she looked happy to see me when I knocked on the door, she was very pleased as Timmy had gone for the whole afternoon and she was lonely, so it all seemed to be going to plan.

She said quite pleasantly for me to move the rubbish off the chair so I could sit down next to her, and she handed me a mug of tea with hardly a half-inch of rim intact. It was the first and last cup of tea my mother ever made me. I'd brought some snacks for us to nibble on, so I drank my by now cold cup of tea and Bridget drank from a can of lager.

I tried to make light conversation but she soon started chatting away, as she so often did, not really letting me get a word in edgeways. I never minded as I was desperate to find out as much information as I could. She was drinking excessively and for a while she fell asleep, so I rushed upstairs to change her bed linen as I brought some new sheets with me.

When she woke up she started on some cans of Breakers, which was Timmy's strong lager which he tried to keep hidden from her. She became more lucid and informative in her conversation, although she rarely finished her sentences. It's as if she had to have a drink first before she could tell me anything from her past. It wasn't so much what she was actually saying, it was the fact that she felt she could talk to me so openly. We were real friends that day. As she became very sleepy again I promised I would come back and see her soon.

I watched her as she closed her eyes, which were grey and sunken in her head. I moved the can from under her cheek and left it by her side. I wished I could tell her who I was. It almost seemed cruel not to, for both of us. As I walked away she extended her hand in a last effort for me to stay but I had to leave. Stephen was expecting me.

It was a cold winter's day towards the end of 1988 when Timmy answered the door, as usual he was in a grumpy mood. He complained he wasn't feeling well and said, 'It's my bleeding chest,' as he lit up a cigarette and inhaled deeply.

I had brought some clothes for Bridget in a carrier bag, which included a thick dressing gown as she always seemed cold despite the fact that the fire was full on. I was worried to ask where she was in case she was back in prison, and Timmy just continued to complain about one thing and another. He shouted, 'Where's my cream mac? It's always hanging on the back of the door and I can't bleeding go out without it.'

Not having any idea where his mac could possibly be, I asked about Bridget. 'Ah,' he shouted, 'she's upstairs, the lazy bitch, she's gone to bed as she said she was cold.'

I hurried upstairs and there was Bridget lying on top of the bed, using Timmy's dirty cream mac as a blanket. She was fast asleep and I hadn't the heart to disturb her, so I went downstairs to make Timmy a cup of tea in an attempt to try to cheer him up.

What I saw as I opened the door really made me laugh. There was Timmy sitting in the lounge in his usual chair, with a fluffy pink dressing gown on. It really did look comical! Even now when I think of it I have to smile.

Bridget's mental state was declining fast, and I knew that I could no longer put off the inevitable. It was a Friday afternoon and I was still calling in to care for my mother and pretending I was there purely on a professional basis. She always addressed me as 'nurse'. We sometimes talked about Phyllis, and I even got used to talking about myself in the third person.

When I knocked on the door Bridget answered, which took me by surprise. I asked, 'Where's Timmy?' She replied rather raucously, 'He's gone into hospital with a bad chest. He's been under the doctor for ages, but the last time he went they took him into the hospital.'

She gave me the impression she thought he was being inconsiderate by going into hospital. I asked how long he had been there. Now irritated by my interest, her voice rose to a higher pitch as she said resentfully, 'I don't know how long he's been in, so why are you asking me?'

I was standing in the lounge. The door to the staircase was ajar. The cream mac that always hung on a hook was there as usual.

Trying to make light conversation, I said, 'Well, at least Timmy won't need his mac while he's in hospital. It's really hot in there.' It was obvious that it was in need of a good wash. It was dirty round the collar, and smelt of cigarettes and greasy food from the fry-ups he often made for himself. Bridget then mumbled something on the lines of, 'Ah, he looks a right old eejit when he wears it. He thinks he's the fecking major in it.' Even though I was feeling apprehensive, I had to smile at her remark.

It was the first time I'd been alone in the house with Bridget for ages, so I seized the opportunity to tell her who I really was. I sat on the same battered chair and peered at my mother's face in the same way as when I'd first met her.

'What would you think if you met Phyllis?' I leant forward to grasp her hand. There was nothing to lose. I decided to come clean and see what reaction I got. I swallowed hard.

'I'm Phyllis, the daughter you gave away all those years ago. Do you remember – you left me at Father Hudson's Homes? I didn't tell you before because I felt it wasn't the right time.'

She stared for a long time and I was relieved that I'd finally told her the truth. But there was no reaction. Not even a glimmer of recognition. I repeated it. She didn't reply but continued to stare.

After a short time she started rambling, as she so often did, talking about trivial things that didn't make any sense. I felt like screaming, but I knew I needed to stay composed.

I was working with patients who had dementia (I still do). I thought, 'My God, I've left it too late.' I knew there never would be a right moment now. I'd lost my mother and found her, but she'd never know.

Even though Bridget was far removed from the longed-for mother figure I'd always hoped to discover,

I still hoped to make a connection with her. It was all the more poignant that she was physically in reach, if not mentally or emotionally. I had cared for my mother from 1981 to 1989 but, as I left her house that afternoon, I kept asking myself, *Why did I leave it so long to tell her?*

Chapter 9

The Nursing Home

It was a long time before I saw my mother again. I was devastated that I had left it too long to tell her that I was her daughter, but I was also going through an entirely separate emotional turmoil. I was pregnant when I told my mother who I was, but I lost the child at the end of 1989. I lost another baby in 1990 when I was almost three months pregnant. So I was so happy when, on 22 September 1991, I gave birth to a healthy boy, called Tom.

In those early days of caring for him, I kept thinking about the special bond a mother has with her child, and I decided I had to call again at my mother's house. I no longer needed to hide behind my disguise as her nurse. The last time I'd visited her I'd told her I was Phyllis, her daughter, but sadly I'd left it too late. She didn't have the mental capacity to take it in, or understand it, so she would never know me as her daughter.

By now it was February 1992 and my two older children were at school. Tom was with his child-minder, so I had the whole day to myself. As I approached Bridget's house I felt as apprehensive as the first time. There was no sign of life, so I stepped back and looked through the window. All was unusually still and quiet. Not the slightest flicker of curtain from next door.

A pile of refuse bags in the corner by the wall in the front garden was bursting open, spilling stale food. This was blending with an overflowing drain to produce a supply of food for more than the local birdlife. I hammered on the door, but it was obvious that the house had been empty for some time.

I had little time to reflect on my findings as a woman's voice reverberated from over the road. 'Nobody's lived there for ages. The last occupants left it in a terrible state.'

A middle-aged woman walked slowly across the road, with her arms folded.

'Do you know what happened to the woman who lived here?' I asked.

'Ah, do you mean that mad Irish woman who was always drunk?'

'Yes,' I said, as she raised her hand to her mouth and clicked her tongue.

'I think …' she paused, as if confirming to herself that she was giving me the right information. 'Yes, I'm almost certain they put her in a nursing home. I know she was in hospital for a long time. She couldn't manage by herself.'

She then went on to give me directions to the local social services office.

'I'm sure they should be able to help you,' she shouted, as I was heading towards the car. Keeping my fingers crossed that she wouldn't ask me any questions, I thanked her for everything and hurried away.

The social services office was only a short drive. I was pleased to find a car parking space at the back, but I thought to myself, *Parking the car is the least of your worries!* I realised that I couldn't pose as my mother's nurse any longer, and that I didn't have my uniform to hide behind. I took a deep breath and walked through the swing doors.

A stern-looking receptionist sat at her desk, but I was surprised and relieved to find there was no queue. 'Can I help you?' she said, before I had time to compose myself.

The waiting area was overflowing with people, and I

needed to speak in confidence to someone, away from prying eyes and wagging ears. I started to explain in a low, soft, hushed voice.

'You will need to speak up, I can't hear you.' I had to be on the ball here so I used the same sharp tone to shout back.

'I've come to see Bridget Ryan's social worker.'

Raising her shoulders and eyebrows a few inches, she said, 'In connection with …?'

'It's a sensitive matter, and I need to speak to her in private,' I replied.

At that point, I wasn't even sure if Bridget had a social worker or, if so, which gender they were. Fortunately she did have an allocated social worker, who was female, so at least it appeared that I was familiar with Bridget's case.

Suddenly I felt more confident. I reminded myself that I'd cared for my mother for eight years after deciding to go it alone, without any help from other professional bodies. I now needed to be confident within my role as Bridget's daughter, but I could draw on my strength as a nurse.

The receptionist seemed to change her attitude and was less intimidating. 'What's your name? Are you a relative of Bridget Ryan?' Without any hesitation I replied, 'Yes, I'm her daughter.'

It just seemed so natural to say and if I'm honest it was almost a relief to be able to tell someone who I really was, albeit not the most sympathetic person. She immediately started to write down my name, then hurried into the back office. I waited for whoever she had to consult to make a decision.

I heard whispering and was conscious that I was being scrutinised. Eventually she returned and asked me to take a seat in the waiting room. 'The social worker will see you shortly,' I was informed.

Making every effort not to trip over feet, mine or other people's, I found one vacant chair in the far corner. After an anxious wait my name was eventually called and I was taken by a tall, slim woman through to a small office at the back of the building. She smiled and introduced herself.

'I'm Frances, Bridget's social worker,' she said, giving me a firm handshake. I thanked her for seeing me at such short notice.

She explained that one of her clients had cancelled their appointment at the last minute, so she had an hour to spare. It was a deprived area of Birmingham, with a lot of social problems, so I'm sure she had a busy case-load. It was as if I was destined to meet her.

'I didn't realise Bridget was in contact with her daughter,' she said, looking bewildered. After offering me a seat she studied me in the same way that the probation officer had done years ago, when I'd first gone in search of my mother.

First I gave her Bridget's date of birth, which confirmed that I was in fact her daughter. Then I enquired about Timmy. She began leafing through Bridget's file, which was on her desk. Looking rather puzzled, she eventually asked, 'Was that the man she lodged with? Ah, he passed away, over two years ago now.' She was not prepared to give me any more details about the circumstances that led to his death, which I realised was due to confidentiality. Although he was a grumpy old man, I was saddened to hear that he'd died.

Although Frances was aware that Bridget had children, she believed they'd all been taken into care years ago, and that she'd never had any contact with any of them. She listened with great interest as I told my story, and assured me that I'd definitely done the right thing by not revealing my true identity.

She was astonished that I'd had the courage to care for my mother, and said that I'd prevented her from going into a home much sooner. I explained how I had become worried, in case I got into trouble for pretending to be Bridget's nurse when in fact I was her natural daughter. She soon put my mind at rest, as she leant over and pressed my shoulder. 'You should be proud of what you did. It's just sad that Bridget suffers from dementia, and will never know.'

Frances explained the circumstances that caused my mother to be taken into a care home. With a big sigh and a sympathetic smile, she clasped her hands together, while resting them on the desk, and looked me straight in the eye. I waited to hear the latest chapter in Bridget's life.

'Your mother was found collapsed and unconscious in an alleyway. It was in the middle of the night and freezing cold, but luckily she was spotted by the police. She was fortunate to have been found, as it was certain that she wouldn't have survived the night.'

She paused. I didn't want to dwell on the fact that my mother would probably have died if she hadn't been found. I think Frances read my mind as she briskly changed her tone.

'Well, that was just over two years ago now. She was rushed into hospital as an emergency, and after some tests she was diagnosed with epilepsy, caused by her alcoholism. She had several seizures while she was in hospital, but eventually, with the right medication, her condition stabilised.'

She stopped briefly, again allowing me time to collect my thoughts. I nodded to acknowledge that she should continue.

'As you are aware, there was a noticeable deterioration in your mother's mental health. She was referred to a psychiatrist, who confirmed that she was suffering from dementia, which I'm sorry to have to say was also associated with alcoholism.'

She wrote down the address and telephone number of the home where my mother was resident, and offered to phone the manager to explain the situation. I appreciated her offer, as it would save me from having to tell the whole story again. She'd been so obliging and I thanked her for all her help. As I left the office she squeezed my hand.

Although I was sad that it had been confirmed that my mother was now suffering from epilepsy — as well as dementia, part of me also felt relieved. At last she was in a safe environment and being looked after by health-care professionals.

I telephoned the care home manager just after 9 a.m. the next day and, as promised, Frances had already given her all the details. Although professional, she was very friendly, and seemed intrigued to meet me.

She said, 'Even though your mother has dementia, she often talks about her children, but doesn't seem to remember their names. Your mother's a real character, although sometimes she can be quite aggressive. It really depends on what type of mood she's in.'

That sounded just like Bridget, I thought! Rather apprehensively, I asked if I could visit my mother later that day. She said I was welcome to visit at any time, and that this was now my mother's home. I thanked her and she said, 'I'm really looking forward to meeting you.' We simultaneously said goodbye, and put down the receiver.

After leaving Tom with his child-minder, I arrived at the home around 11 a.m. It was only a short distance from where she'd previously lived, so at least I was familiar with the area. It was a fairly new, purpose-built care home. I felt extremely anxious at the prospect of seeing my mother after such a long time, and I suppose I was also worried about meeting the staff who were looking after her, as it certainly was an unusual case.

There were plenty of spaces in the large car park in front of the home, and I sat there for some time gathering my thoughts before entering the building.

This was going to be the first time I'd visited my mother as her daughter, and in such a public place. I quickly reminded myself of how I'd dealt with bathing my mother in her drunken stupor; how I'd coped with Timmy's hostile, often threatening, behaviour. But that was now all in the past.

I rang the doorbell and a woman in a light green uniform opened the door. As I stepped inside, I was greeted with a welcoming smile. However, she appeared confused when I told her, 'I've come to see Bridget Ryan.' Looking extremely puzzled, she said, 'But Bridget never has any visitors.'

I squeezed past her, my heart thumping as I said, 'Um, um, I've got an appointment with the manager.' Thankfully I was soon rescued, as the manager walked towards me, with her arms open, enfolding me in a warm embrace.

'Hello, you must be Phyllis?' she said, telling me her name was Lisa.

Realising how nervous I was, she asked, 'Would you like a nice cup of tea?' and led me into her office, which helped me feel less conspicuous. Lisa then asked a member of staff for a pot of tea for two, adding, 'I don't want any interruptions, so if anybody phones, just ask them to ring back later.'

I started to relax, and leant back in one of the comfortable chairs in her office. She had Bridget's care plan on her lap. It was like she was hugging it. I couldn't help but speculate what an interesting read it would be, as Bridget was certainly a unique person. After a few minutes there was a knock on the door. This time it was a much younger woman who brought in the tea and biscuits. I suspected that she was also curious to see what Bridget's daughter actually looked like.

There was an uncomfortable moment of silence as Lisa glanced at me. I imagine she was looking for any similarity between me and Bridget. She quickly turned her head and apologised, while offering me a biscuit, almost as a distraction. Then she set about explaining some points about my mother's condition.

'I realise that Frances has already given you the

background information about the circumstances that led to your mother requiring full-time care. However, I'll explain a few more details, if that's OK?' As she opened the care plan, which was still balanced on her lap, I listened attentively to the latest instalment of my mother's life.

'Your mother has been a resident here for almost two years now. She was admitted on 20 June 1990. She had been in hospital for a long time. When the man she lodged with died, she needed to go into a home, as she could never have coped by herself. At that time she had no known relatives.'

Conscious that her remark may have caused me some distress, she quickly added, 'Frances told me how you'd nursed your mother at home for eight years, without her even realising who you were. That must have been so hard for you.' Not really knowing how to reply to her question, I just smiled.

Lisa continued to tell me about my mother's behaviour. It certainly appeared that she was quite challenging at times. She then showed me a photograph of Bridget when she'd been taken out for the day. It made me feel very emotional. Although she looked older, her face was much fatter, she looked well groomed, and she'd even had her hair brushed for the occasion. The sad thing was, although she was now living with dementia, she looked more normal in that photograph than I'd ever seen her look before.

Lisa left the office for a few minutes while she arranged for Bridget to be taken into a small lounge further along the corridor. When she came back she explained, 'Bridget has her own bedroom, at the back of the building.' I thought to myself, at least she's got some privacy, as some of the residents did have shared rooms, but it was soon made clear to me that the main reason Bridget needed a single room was because she had become so disruptive, especially during the night.

Apparently she often screamed, and could sometimes be aggressive towards the other residents for no particular reason. She sometimes lashed out at the staff, was unpredictable, and couldn't be trusted.

Well, that was Lisa's summary of Bridget's behaviour. I realised that she needed to tell me the problems they'd been faced with. It just made me feel sad, as during our conversation she'd informed me that Bridget no longer drank alcohol. In fact, she'd forgotten that she was ever dependent on it. This was very poignant. The thing that had damaged my mother's brain, and contributed to her living the life that she had, she didn't crave anymore. But because of it, I'd lost the mother I had finally found.

'Well, Phyllis, are you ready to see your mother?'

I nodded.

Lisa clarified the arrangements. 'It will be better if we use the small lounge. It's quieter in there. Most of the relatives like to use this lounge, especially if they want to have a natter with their loved ones without being disturbed. It's so much better than the communal lounge – it's not very private there, as there are usually lots of different conversations going on at the same time.'

She continued in a matter-of-fact way, as if I was just an ordinary relative. 'When you've had a chat with your mum, I'll show you her bedroom and then I can give you a tour of the home.' But how else did I expect her to act?

I felt confused and very anxious. It was like meeting my mother for the first time all over again. The only difference was that I could now call her Mum but, regrettably, she wouldn't know. Lisa gave me a friendly wink, and said she would now let me have some time alone with my mother.

I made my way towards the small lounge, gingerly opening the door, and feeling scared of what was behind it. There was my mother, sitting on the sofa, just staring out of the window. She turned, but there was no recognition, no facial expression, only her wide, gaping eyes. It was as if a complete stranger had just entered the room.

I was aching to say, *Hello, Mum, it's Phyllis, your long-lost daughter,* but my mouth was dry, I just couldn't say a word. As I sat beside her on the sofa, clutching her hand, I noticed that she now had clean, manicured fingernails. Tears started rolling down my face.

I managed to retrieve a tissue from my bag, trying desperately to hide the fact that I was crying. Suddenly there was a tap on the door. It was a relief to see Lisa's friendly face peeping around the door, and she immediately saw that I was upset. She said, 'Bridget's just had her medication, so I'm sure that's why she's not responding to you.' It just looked as if she was in a world of her own, and totally unaware of her surroundings.

After a while, Lisa gave me the promised tour of the home. It was obvious that there were other residents with dementia. Some chatted to me as if I were their long lost friend, yet my own mother hadn't spoken a word to me.

As we walked into the bedroom it was sparsely furnished; no ornaments or pictures of any description.

Lisa must have read my mind, and told me why the bedroom was so spartan. 'As I pointed out earlier, your mother can often be aggressive, and she's been known to throw things. She broke the mirror on her dressing table the other day, so it had to be removed. She really can't be trusted.'

I sneaked a look in her wardrobe, and it was almost empty with only a few items of clothing. Lisa said, 'You're welcome to bring in any photographs, perhaps one of yourself? If it's framed, we can get the handyman to put it on the wall.'

I decided this was not a good idea. First, she was likely to have thrown something at it, but second, and more importantly, she wouldn't have any recollection of me as her daughter, so it would be meaningless.

We went back into Lisa's office for a chat before I left. I'd already made my mind up that it was best if I didn't go back to see Bridget that day. I just didn't want to make a scene; I already felt self-conscious and had the impression that I was the talk of the home. It seemed that most of the staff were curious to see what Bridget's long-lost daughter really looked like.

Lisa asked, 'Would you like to meet your mother's GP? She will be able to give you more details of her medical condition. After all, you are her next of kin, and you have a right to know.' It was the first time I'd ever thought about it, and it did feel a bit weird. I said I would be pleased to meet her, so Lisa telephoned and made an appointment for the following Saturday at midday.

Dr Watkins apparently told Lisa that she would have finished surgery by then, so we would have more time to talk. I was grateful that she was prepared to see me, and I thanked Lisa for all her help.

She gave me Dr Watkins' phone number and the surgery's address, and advised me to give her a call before I went, just to make sure she hadn't been called out on an emergency. Lisa suddenly remembered that she hadn't got my address or telephone number. As she started to write it in Bridget's care plan she hesitated and said, 'Ah, it will be nice to fill in the blank space by "next of kin".' Her pen hovered as she asked, 'Will it be all right to put you down as Bridget's daughter?'

I thought about it for a few moments and then replied, 'Well I suppose I am, so why not? Just don't put all the details about me being adopted as it will just complicate things.' I had spent my life keeping my adoption a secret, so I thought it was simpler not to put it in writing now. However, it did cause complications later, as some of the staff didn't realise how unusual our relationship was. But more of that later.

I left the home feeling emotionally exhausted. I collected Tom from the child minder, giving him the biggest cuddle ever, and went home for a cup of tea, realising how important being part of a family really is.

The following Saturday morning I telephoned the surgery and asked if I could speak to Dr Watkins. To my surprise she answered the phone.

I quickly blurted out, 'I'm Bridget Ryan's daughter. The manager of her care home made an appointment for me to see you this morning.'

She said, 'Yes, that will be fine. Just come along at midday as arranged,' and the line went dead. I'd been feeling relatively calm, but I was now apprehensive as she almost seemed dismissive of me, as if I were being a nuisance. I only hoped she'd be more welcoming when I met her.

Dr Watkins was the designated GP for the home, and visited most Thursday mornings. Bridget had only been her patient from when she was admitted into the home. As I walked towards the reception area, a more approachable receptionist, a little flustered, greeted me with a warm smile.

'Hello, have you come to see Dr Watkins?' she asked. Before I had time to answer her she said, 'If you'd like to go through to consulting room 4, Dr Watkins is waiting to see you.' She gave me the impression that she'd been well informed about my visit.

There was no time to gather my thoughts which, in hindsight, was probably for the best. I thanked her and headed towards room 4. On entering I coughed nervously and Dr Watkins joked, 'You should see a doctor about that cough,' which helped break the ice. She seemed totally different now in person.

'Sit yourself down, I don't bite,' she said, immediately reminding me of my meeting with Miss McFadden at the orphanage.

We were both aware that there was no need for any introductions, as I knew Lisa had filled her in with all the details. I felt relaxed in her company and was happy to answer any of her questions. I was eager to ask her a few too. She leant back in her chair, with her hands clasped, resting on her lap, but did not stare in the same way that everyone else had done previously.

'What made you decide to trace your mother?' she asked.

'Curiosity got the better of me,' I replied. 'I'd always been told as a child that my natural parents had both died of TB.'

She paused and thought for a moment while she digested what I had said.

'When you're adopted you have a right to be told the truth. You need to know if there's any history of genetic disorders or inherited diseases.' I nodded in agreement.

There was a small box on her desk containing medical cards which she rifled through to find Bridget's notes. I was surprised that it wasn't as full as I'd expected. Taking into account her past medical history, her complex needs and present condition, I imagined her notes to be bulging.

Dr Watkins explained that the notes only went to 1958. My heart missed a beat as I leant across and noticed on a small medical card: Given birth to a healthy baby girl, 8lbs 2oz at Gulson Hospital in Coventry on 26 May 1959. Normal delivery. Baby and mother doing well.

I shouted excitedly, 'That must be me. Is that how much I weighed?'

Dr Watkins was looking a little puzzled and asked, 'What year were you born?' She realised that I'd got mixed up, and explained, 'That was your mother's second daughter, Angela.'

Of course – the date hadn't registered. I was born in 1956. Angela was born three years later. For a moment I felt very disappointed. Yet again, there was no documentation that my mother had ever given birth to me. Dr Watkins soon cleared up the confusion, and explained that my mother's medical notes had been lost when she changed her surname to Ryan.

'It must have been an awful shock for you to discover that your mother was a down-and-out,' said the doctor.

I was a little unsettled by her description, so I paused to collect my thoughts. 'I know what I found wasn't exactly a perfect mother, but I don't regret tracing her, and I'm glad that I found her. It's the sort of nightmare all adopted people dread when they go in search of their mother, isn't it?' I replied.

'Although what I found wasn't good, it's a terrible feeling to know you have a mother somewhere out there, but you don't know who, or what, or where. You don't know where you come from, or who you are, or what happened to you that made your mother give you away. There should be more honesty all along in adoptions: no secrets, no mysteries. I'd rather know the worst than nothing at all.'

Dr Watkins appeared to sympathise with what I was saying, and commented on how well I appeared to be coping. 'It's a good job you have such a strong character. Perhaps for another adopted person finding a mother like that might have done more harm than good. I'll give you as much information as I can, although some of the details are rather vague and not too reliable.'

Now it was her turn to look confused, which wasn't surprising as the medical card was rather contradictory. After Bridget's original case notes had been lost, she gave the doctor at the time her past medical history. Knowing her, I think she may have deliberately tried to baffle the medical profession, and had tried to cover up her previous mistakes.

Dr Watkins was extremely helpful, and wrote down the information she had, for me to take away. 'Well, I can only tell you what's in front of me, but how much of it is true I don't honestly know.' She reassured me that there were no inherited conditions for me to be worried about. Her epilepsy and dementia were caused by her alcoholism.

Then she went on to tell me the birthdates of my half-siblings, although it still seemed rather muddled. There were three children born after me. Two were brought up together in foster care and the last was adopted.

It was a lot to take in. I was very preoccupied by my mother's condition of course. As much as I could think about my half siblings, it seemed cruel to trace them just to tell them about what their mother was like today. I hoped they had had happy lives. Who was I to disrupt them? It could have done more harm than good. Dr Watkins said she felt I was coping well with the situation and that I was very self-reliant.

Over the next year I visited my mother about once a month, usually on a Sunday morning as it was much quieter. I never really enjoyed the visits. I suppose it was more out of duty than anything else, and I always came away feeling upset.

I took her the new clothes and toiletries that she clearly needed, but as I'd been advised not to take in any ornaments, her bedroom remained very much the same as I'd first seen it. At least she had some new clothes to wear and smelt nicer.

I sometimes helped the carers give my mother a shower if she became aggressive towards them, but it was something I found increasingly tough to do. It was difficult to be her nurse any longer. Seeing her in a state of undress, she was so frail, the years and the alcohol had taken their toll. I wanted to step back from being her nurse and openly be her daughter. But sadly I could never do it the way I wanted to because of her dementia.

Most of the staff in the home were friendly, but one or two of the carers did appear a little hostile towards me. I think they had come to their own conclusions, not knowing that I was adopted and had only traced my mother when I was an adult because it wasn't in her care plan. The relationship I had had with my mother was not going to be the same as if she had brought me up, yet, strangely enough, I had cared for my mother in a way that most daughters would never have to. I can honestly say our relationship was unique.

I reminded myself that I had come to visit my mother and I shouldn't feel that I have to justify myself to different staff every time I visited. I tried not to think about their attitude towards me. It is so easy to judge someone without knowing the full facts. It certainly gave me a much greater understanding of how difficult it is when a loved one is living with dementia. I now have genuine empathy with relatives when they are visiting loved ones in the care home where I now work.

One morning, when Tom was about 18 months old, I was off from work and hadn't decided what to do. Stuart and Hannah had just gone back to school after the Easter holidays, and I was getting Tom ready to take him out for a few hours before lunch. At this point I had not decided where to go. It was a cold, rainy day, so I knew it needed to be somewhere indoors.

I was sitting on the floor next to Tom in the lounge, building a tower with his wooden bricks. He thought it was great fun to knock them down again, clapping his hands and shouting 'Yeah!' at the top of his voice. It always gave me such a warm glow to see his face light up with such pleasure.

At times like that my mother would often come into my thoughts, and I was saddened to think that she never had such memories of her own children. Suddenly I said, 'I know what we can do today. Shall we visit your grandmother?' I remember Tom shouting back 'Yeah!' because he'd just knocked down the second tower of bricks I'd only just finished building.

However, he'd answered my question, and I suddenly realised that she'd never met any of her grandchildren. It somehow seemed the right thing to do. I realised that Tom was too young to remember the occasion so, if things didn't turn out as planned, it wasn't going to upset him at all. I felt I had nothing to lose, and at least I would have Tom with me for some moral support – sometimes the visits seemed so meaningless, as she never knew who I was.

We arrived at the home just before lunchtime. There was now an intercom by the front door, so I pressed the red button and spoke through the mouth piece. I said, 'I've come to visit Bridget Ryan.' I immediately felt relieved, for I recognised Lisa's voice as she instructed me to push the door open. She gave me her usual welcoming smile, and of course was excited to meet Tom, who was enjoying all the attention.

I wheeled his pushchair into the small lounge as Lisa had suggested. She asked one of the carers standing in the corridor to bring Bridget in so she could 'meet her lovely grandson'. I started feeling apprehensive in case she became aggressive towards him, but Lisa reassured me and said, 'Your mother is more manageable these days. Some of her medication has been changed, and she seems much calmer. Well, as long as she's got her cigarettes, that is.'

In the distance I could hear some shouting and then, recognising that distinctive Tipperary accent, I knelt down to reassure Tom, as by now he was becoming a little fidgety. I said, 'Can you hear your noisy grandmother?' I took him out of his pushchair and squeezed him tightly, which comforted me as much as him, and headed towards the sofa. I could hear Bridget shouting as she walked in.

'Ah, Jaysus Christ I want a cigarette.' Lisa was also not far behind, and doing her best to persuade Bridget that it wasn't such a good idea to be smoking around a small child, but she was far from convinced.

'Jaysus, will you just give me a bleeding cigarette? The little boy isn't going to be bothered with me smoking,' she said. She was duly given some Park Drive cigarettes.

With all the commotion I hadn't had time to reflect on Tom's first meeting with his grandmother. He seemed more than happy exploring his new environment, and wasn't disturbed by his grandmother's noisy expletives.

Lisa had arranged a tray of tea. As expected, my mother soon calmed down when she'd had her cigarette. She sat next to me on the sofa and started to stare at Tom. I felt overwhelmed by the whole experience. She was staring at her grandson, but sadly she would never really know him.

After a few minutes I looked into her eyes and said, 'Say hello to your grandson.' If only for a split second there seemed a glimpse of recognition in her face. I held her hand and emphasised, 'This is Tom, your grandson.' She smiled and continued staring at him for a while and then in a caring way – a side to my mother I'd never seen before – she said so tenderly, 'He's a beautiful little baby.' Within minutes I had lost that moment, but it was one I will treasure forever.

Suddenly she looked scared. It's hard to explain, but it was as if she had switched off all her emotions. Instead of the alcohol causing the communication block, it was now her dementia. Her expression just completely changed. Tom, with his blonde hair, was very like me as a child. Maybe it had triggered some memories that she'd rather not think about.

Within minutes she was like a totally different person, acting very bossy and shouting, 'Why isn't he at school?' I tried to explain that he wasn't even two years old yet, but she wasn't listening and just started to ramble, as she so often did. I had to smile to myself. There was my own mother telling me how to look after my son, when she herself had been far from ideal.

Tom then moved one of the cushions on the sofa and she started shouting at the top of her voice, 'Put it down!' She made him jump, as she had such a piercing voice, and he started crying. I'm sure she frightened him to death. To my annoyance she then started mimicking him. 'Ah, he's a cry-baby.' I picked him up to comfort him and she shouted, 'Leave him, leave him.'

Her horrible words rang in my head. 'Leave him, leave him.' I felt so angry. I wanted to shout back at her, like you left me when I was crying as a baby.

By now I wasn't thinking rationally. It was the first time I'd felt such anger towards her and I needed to leave with Tom. I'd lost the mother I had found, so why did I think things would be any different with her as a grandmother? At least I'd tried. The one thing I was certain about was that I wouldn't be taking Tom to visit her again.

As we left the home I whispered into Tom's ear, still smelling the cigarette smoke on his little head, 'Say goodbye to your grandmother.' It was so poignant to see his little hand waving goodbye to a grandmother he would never know.

Chapter 10

Her Final Years

Over the next eight years I visited my mother a few times a year. At Christmas and on her birthday I always took a card, but never one with the word 'mother' on. It's hard to explain, but it wouldn't have felt right. She never knew me as her daughter, so I was more at ease with sending her a card for 'someone special' which, in spite of all that had happened, is what she was to me.

Sometimes I visited her in the spring because it's such an optimistic time. It was always emotional, invariably I would come away feeling upset. By now my mother was at the end stage of dementia, and often could be very aggressive. I was also busy bringing up my own children and I needed to make sure that the impact of visiting her wasn't going to affect them in any way.

At least I knew she was safe and being well looked after. I'd often phone the home to ask how she was getting on. Usually I was told something along the lines of, 'She's fine, no change in her condition.' This didn't give me a great deal of comfort, but at least I knew she was still alive and kicking. Literally, in her case.

My mother usually sat in the small day room with another resident called Rose, who also had dementia, although not as advanced as my mother's. She was never physically aggressive towards Rose. They'd often sit together for hours, smoking and chatting, clearly not remembering what the other had said. But they were good friends and seemed to enjoy each other's company.

It was quite amusing to watch them together. One minute they'd be pouring out a torrent of abuse, blaming each other for the argument, but within minutes they'd forgotten it and were the best of friends again. I was glad that my mother had made one friend who she could chat to, or at least argue with.

In 1996, Tom was in nursery and Hannah had joined Stuart at secondary school. District nursing was changing. Computers were coming in, we had to log our times and mileage, and the job was becoming more stressful.

I loved visiting patients in their own home, but now we didn't have as much time to spend with them and I decided I needed to have a career change, so I left the district and started working in care homes. But I made sure I avoided my mother's home. I was Phyllis now, not her nurse.

My mother's health continued to decline. It was August 2001 when I visited her for the last time, although I wasn't aware that it would be the last scene of our complicated relationship.

It had been almost a year since my last visit, but the sun was shining and I was in a pleasant frame of mind.

That was to be short-lived. I arrived to a hostile reception when I informed the carer, 'I'm Bridget Ryan's daughter.' She seemed irritated by my visit. 'She's still in bed,' she replied.

She led me into the dining room where it was quieter, as the other residents were sitting in the communal lounge. Not even bothering to introduce herself – I'd never met her before – she instructed me to wait in the dining room until they got her up. She continued talking as she cleared away the breakfast dishes from the table. I felt that she deliberately made no eye contact.

'Your mother's been a real pain, shouting and screaming for most of the night, disturbing all the other residents and causing such trouble for everyone.'

Before I had a chance to reply, she left the dining room, making absolutely sure she had closed the doors firmly behind her. I was alone with a TV programme that no one was watching. My mood dipped dramatically. Perhaps I had a premonition of what was to come. I felt like running away and never going back, but I wanted to see how my mother was getting on as it had been almost a year since I'd last seen her.

I suddenly heard a commotion. I turned my head to look, and there was my mother flailing about in her wheelchair, being pushed through the double doors by the carer-with-no-name.

She looked very frail and had lost a lot of weight. As a nurse, caring for patients with dementia, I knew the right questions to ask, but no words came out. In my head I wanted to ask: *Why is she in a wheelchair? Is she now immobile? Why has she lost so much weight? Is she not eating very much? Why does she look so frail? Has her condition deteriorated? Why is she not sleeping at night? Can't she be prescribed some medication to help her sleep?* There were so many 'whys', and I probably knew the answer to all of them.

But it's different when it's your own mother. You seem to forget all the things you know. I often have to answer relatives' questions and give them reassurance. I suppose I needed some reassurance myself that day.

Bridget had been wheeled to a big round table in the corner of the room and two trollies appeared outside the door. I was handed a lidded plastic beaker which I assumed had tea in it. I moved it towards her mouth, but she shifted her head away and kept her teeth clamped shut. I desperately tried to give her a few sips.

A different carer, whose voice was much kinder, and whom I recognised from one of my previous visits, came over and said, 'Your mother isn't drinking much these days.' How ironic, I thought. If only I'd been told that when I'd first met her almost 20 years ago, things could have been very different. But of course it was tea we were talking about now, not alcohol.

I sat for some time, holding my mother's hands. She spoke infrequently and when she did, it made little sense. Her words gradually became a babble, often screaming, as before. I smiled and tried to make some kind of connection, but she had such anger in her face and seemed so tormented.

To my horror, she became extremely aggressive

towards me, shouting and digging her fingernails into my wrist. It was really hurting, but I just couldn't escape her grasp. Her eyes were wide open and she looked like a woman possessed, grinding her stained nicotine teeth and using all her strength to dig further into my skin. I felt the tears rolling down my face as I screamed in sheer disbelief. We were alone in the dining room; there was nobody to come to my rescue, and the pain from my wrist became unbearable.

Why did my mother want to hurt me so much? I was in such agony, emotionally and physically, but I mustered all the strength I could and eventually managed to escape from her grip. My wrist throbbed with pain and started to bleed, and the marks of her nails stayed on my skin. I didn't want to hate my mother, but I was upset and hurting. I felt shocked and completely powerless. I'd dealt with aggressive residents on many occasions, but this situation was different. I desperately wanted to detach myself from what had just happened.

After all, my mother had dementia and wasn't aware of what she was doing. I hung on for a moment until I regained control.

I've tried so many times to remember what I did actually say to the carer-with-no-name as I left my mother for the last time. Still severely shocked after my mother's attack, I asked to see the manager. I was told, 'She's not here on Sundays, so if you've got a problem you will need to speak to me.' I blurted out something along the lines of, 'I think it's best if I don't visit my mother any more. I just can't cope with her aggression. I don't want to hate her, so it's better if I stay away. If she's really ill, then phone me.'

What she thought about my outburst I can only imagine, but I realise now how much I'd been misunderstood on that day. The anonymous carer clearly wasn't aware of the circumstances, or that I'd been adopted. If she had known the effort I'd made to find my mother, she'd know that I'd never have wanted to sever all connection with her.

Whatever was written in my mother's care plan that day inevitably led to the mix-up that followed, and to why I never saw her again. I remember very clearly my mother's tormented face as I walked away that last time. It is something I deeply regret, as it was to be the last image I had of her, and to this day it remains etched in my memory. All I ever wanted was for her to find some peace and happiness before she died. I didn't look back as I hurried out of the home. Sitting in my car with a heavy heart, and sobbing uncontrollably, I knew I'd reached the end of the line.

Over the next 18 months I often telephoned the home to enquire how my mother was getting on. I was always told the same. 'She's fine, no real change in her condition.'

I shall never forget the night of 17 February 2003. I was at home with my youngest son, Tom, who was by then 11. About 9 p.m. the telephone rang. I rushed to answer it.

'Hello …?'

An unexpectedly sharp voice on the other end of the line demanded, 'Can I speak to Bridget Ryan's daughter?'

Feeling a little startled, I said, 'Er, yes. Speaking.'

Not giving me a moment to collect my thoughts she blurted out, 'Just to let you know your mother's passed away.'

My voice cracking, I asked incredulously, 'Why wasn't I kept up to date about her health deteriorating?'

Her cold, disapproving reply shook me to the core. 'It's written clearly in her notes: daughter only wants to be contacted in the event of her mother's death.'

'Why was she admitted to hospital? How long has she been there?'

'Your mother was with us for three weeks. She came in with dehydration and a chest infection, which inevitably led to pneumonia, which was the main cause of her death. Dementia was the secondary cause.'

Not one mention of her alcoholism – it was almost as if she'd been teetotal all her life. Her death was such a shock. It didn't help that the woman on the other end of the line dismissed my attempts to explain why I was not there at her bedside. I said there must have been some misunderstanding when I gave my instructions to the home. I had asked to be told if her condition worsened, and that hadn't happened. But nothing was going to shake this woman's belief in my apparent lack of interest. Her opinion shouldn't have mattered, but after my complicated history with my mother it really hurt.

Thinking about it now I still feel very cross. As a nurse myself, I believe it is part of our role to comfort and care in times of need.

She gave me the number of a social worker who was dealing with my mother's case, and the rest of the conversation remains a blur. When I put the phone down, if I had to sum up my feelings in three words they would be: stunned, tearful, angry.

It was inevitable that one day her death would come, but the woman's tone was so mean. I felt bewildered as to why she told me in such a cruel way. I desperately hoped that my mother's life had ended with some degree of dignity, which unfortunately she had been denied when she was alive, and that her death was tranquil.

Tom looked puzzled. 'Why are you crying, Mum?' he asked. Then realisation hit – I hadn't told him I had been adopted. There had never been any point, because what would have been the benefit? Yet it now felt wrong, morally wrong. His own flesh and blood, his grandmother, had just died and he didn't even know of her existence.

I had told my two older children, although they'd never known the circumstances. How could I have ever introduced my children to such a grandmother?

I shook my head, conscious of how closely I was being scrutinised. Before I had time to gather my thoughts I found myself telling him a blatant lie. 'Work has just phoned. One of the residents at the nursing home has just passed away.'

His expression suggested that he wasn't convinced. 'You wouldn't be this upset, Mum. Who's really died?' I'd never envisaged having to tell him in this way, but he was so sensitive to my emotions.

As he sat beside me on the sofa, I started to explain. 'I have something to tell you that I haven't mentioned before. You know how some people are adopted ...' and I went on to tell him about my mother.

He seemed partly relieved because at first he thought I was about to tell him that he had been adopted. I quickly reassured him that in fact it was me, and he listened attentively to the whole story. He was amazed when I told him that he had actually met his grand-mother when he was 18 months old, but obviously he had been too young to remember that.

Children are much more resilient than we realise. He didn't seem upset by what I told him; he wasn't emo-tionally involved, so he was able to adjust easily.

'Good night, Mum. I love you,' he said on his way to bed. Putting his mind at rest I told him, 'I'm fine, and I love you, too.'

Close to midnight, with sleep eluding me, I tried to make sense of things. Don't we all live life for the simple desire to be happy? My mother had never stood a chance. I hoped that now she was at peace.

Because of her past it seemed a merciful release, and there were now no loose ends. But it was so final, and I grieved for a mother who never knew me as her daughter. Sometimes death can be neat and tidy, and fit into place like the last piece of a jigsaw. Although at times I was troubled by finding such a dysfunctional mother, I'm so glad I did. She was the last piece of my own jigsaw.

A few days passed before I summoned up the courage to telephone the number the nurse had given me. A cheerful man with a distinctive Irish accent answered my call.

'Can I speak to Michael Dwyer, please?'

'Speaking.'

'My name's Phyllis. It's about my mother, Bridget Ryan.

'Ah, I'm so glad you called, I've been thinking about you. I'm Bridget's appointed social worker and I'll be helping you make the funeral arrangements. I'd like to convey my condolences on the loss of your mother, who I believed you nursed for many years, without her ever knowing you were her daughter.'

I was touched by his kindness, and was relieved that

the nursing home seemed to have passed on the full story this time.

'It may take several weeks for the funeral to be arranged. I need to sort out your mother's affairs. She had some money in a building society account, which I'm sure she'd forgotten.'

He wasn't certain of the amount, or if it was enough to cover all the funeral costs, but he reassured me that he'd keep me informed of any further developments. I put the phone down, feeling that a great weight had been lifted from my shoulders. I knew then that I wasn't alone and that he was there to support me.

As promised, a few weeks later he phoned, and told me that my mother had enough in her account to ensure that she would be able to have a respectable funeral – although of course that was something I would have always made sure of.

So, while she rested at the funeral parlour and all the arrangements were being made, I consulted my diary and decided that the second week in March would be a suitable date for her funeral.

I telephoned the funeral directors to arrange for a wreath to be placed on my mother's coffin. They asked if I wanted any special message written on the card. It was only then that I was able to say, 'Please write: To Mum with love from your nurse, who was your daughter Phyllis, and your grandchildren send their love x.'

My daughter Hannah was now 18, and had arranged to have the day off from work so she could give me some much-needed moral support.

We left the house with time to spare before my mother's coffin was due to pass the care home, where she'd spent the last 13 years of her life. I will always be grateful to Hannah for the thoughtfulness and sensitivity that she showed me on that difficult day.

'Let's have a quick half, in memory of Nan,' Hannah said. We had spotted the run-down pub on the corner, near the care home. I recognised it as the pub she frequently drank in more than 20 years ago, when I'd first met her. It seemed quite fitting to do something like that. After all, I'm sure it was where she'd spent a lot of her time.

As we stepped inside our feet stuck to the carpet. The air tasted like a damp sock, hitting the back of my throat so hard I started to cough, which only made us more conspicuous as we walked to the bar to order our drinks.

The appearance of strangers aroused interest and the locals muttered to each other at the other side of the bar.

As we looked over we noticed a few furtive glances, and then unashamed stares. We raised and clinked our glasses, 'Cheers to Tipperary Mary. God bless her,' we said in unison.

Realising the time, we hurried across the road where the funeral car was waiting. The hearse had already left, as we'd spent too much time in the pub, which somehow seemed fitting. Hannah joked, 'Nan would be proud of us.'

It was a low-key affair, with the five-strong congregation travelling together in one funeral car. There was Hannah and me, and a carer from the home that I didn't know, but who seemed a very gentle type of girl. She was escorting Rose, my mother's one and only friend.

Last was Sister Katherine, with whom I struck up an instant rapport. She was calm and kind, but delightfully eccentric. She knew my mother very well and had visited the home every Friday afternoon when she tried to give her Holy Communion but was always told to 'clear off' by my mother. With a little giggle she said, 'Well she used the "F" word but it's best if I don't use that sort of language as I am a nun. Ah, but she wasn't of sound mind and God will absolve her of all her sins.'

Sister Katherine gave me a sympathy card, which she wrote on the way to the crematorium. She asked me my daughter's name so that she could include her, which was so thoughtful.

Although my mother's passing was tinged with sadness, there were comic moments thanks to lovely Rose, who was such a lively character. Because of her condition her short-term memory was poor, so she was constantly asking the same questions.

'Has someone died?' she kept asking, before bursting into tears, as if it was the first time she'd heard the sad news that it was Bridget who'd died. Rose wept a little and sang a little, although she couldn't always remember why she was crying.

During the journey she seemed to be in a trance, as if in deep thought, and then she leant forward and whispered, 'What was it that killed her exactly? Did I know her?' Sister Katherine replied, 'Yes, she was your dear friend, but she was sick.'

Although Rose also had dementia, she sometimes

had lucid moments. Suddenly she said, 'Ah it's funny Bridget going like that, and she's still got some of my fags!' This caused such laughter while we were on the way to the crematorium that it must have looked a little strange to onlookers.

But then my mother's funeral – and her whole life – was anything but normal.

I began to feel apprehensive as we approached the entrance of the crematorium and saw the hearse draw up at the gates. It seemed almost odd for her to have such a tidy, respectable and conventional end to her life.

I caught sight of my mother's coffin. I needed to show respect, but I know an onlooker would not have thought I looked sad. Maybe part of me felt relief.

As she was carried into the chapel I thought of how I knew as a child that she was still alive somewhere, even though my adoptive mother had always insisted she was dead. I knew my story wouldn't have a fairy-tale ending, but I never regretted finding her. We all have a right to know who we are and where we come from. I was able to look after her for eight years, without her knowing I was her daughter. When I did tell her it was too late, but I hoped she could now rest in peace.

***

Walking into the empty chapel really tugged at my heartstrings. I often attend residents' funerals from the nursing home where I work, and the crematorium is usually full to capacity. But my mother's passing had gone almost unnoticed by the outside world.

I tried not to dwell on that for too long. Did it really matter? My mother would never know who did or didn't go to her funeral.

The organ played 'Abide with Me' and the undertaker standing in the doorway did his best to conceal a smile as Rose sang at the top of her voice. She didn't know the words and was totally out of tune, but I was so glad she was there that day.

My eyes still stayed dry. I felt as though I was watching it all from the outside. I muttered prayers under my breath. There were a few suitably solemn hymns that I hadn't even been asked about, but I cleared my throat in an attempt to hum the tune. Again Rose came to my rescue, singing loudly, although it was a different hymn. I smile as I think of it now.

Then the priest started talking about my mother and I realised he had no idea of the type of person she really was, and the heartache she'd had. He was talking about the woman who had brought me into the world, but who had been denied the joy of ever being a real mother. It was only then that I felt tears running down my face.

Epilogue

The two mothers who shaped my life truly believed they had my interests at heart. Bridget handed me over to the orphanage to save me from her dysfunctional life; my adoptive mother gave me stability and in her own clumsy way protected me from the truth.

I actually grew closer to my adoptive mother in her later years. Stephen and I drifted apart and separated in 2004. We divorced the following year. Both my adoptive parents helped out with Tom, who was still young at 13. I'd leave Tom with Dad, while I went shopping with Mum, coming home for one of Dad's teas.

When Dad died from a stroke in 2007, Mum went to pieces. She'd never had to pay bills before, and she had no one to boss about! I also realised she was showing signs of dementia. I visited her most days on my way to work and took her for a trip out when I could. Often she'd cover up how ill she was. Mum had always wanted to appear respectable and she would have hated people to know that she had dementia. What was touching was that she sometimes let her guard down, saying things to me like, 'Oh your hair looks nice' or 'Thank you for helping, I'd be lost without you'. Things she'd never said before. In her final years, because of my nursing skills, at last my mother valued and respected me as her trusted daughter.

In July 2013 she went into hospital, and a few months later died in my arms. I feel privileged to have had that time with her to say goodbye. Five days later my first grandchildren were born – Hannah's twin girls, Isabelle and Emmy. It was so special to have the opportunity to meet my birth mother, and to love and care for her. At her funeral, when I said goodbye, I promised one day I would tell our story.

Mum, I hope I've done you proud…

Acknowledgements

This book would not have happened without the help and support of Barbara Fisher. We first met when I was nursing her dear mother, Nora Parsons, who had dementia. I was with Barbara when her mother passed away which brought us closer together. We continued to meet up regularly and she was a huge help to me writing this book. She is one special lady! I'd also like to thank her husband, Mike, who was very supportive!

I'd like to thank all of the staff, residents and relatives at Neville Williams Nursing Home (past and present). Who gave me encouragement and followed me on my journey.

My friends in Kefalonia, Greece who have been so supportive while I was writing my book. I have enjoyed many lovely times there and hope to have many more in the future.

I'm grateful to everyone who helped me on the journey to finding my birth mother, especially John the social worker and Bernadette her probation officer, who really did have a soft spot for Tipperary Mary. I'd like to thank them for their information, support and direction. Thanks also to Charlotte Cole, Jo Sollis and the Mirror Books team for their help and advice.

Thank you to my three lovely children, my daughter's partner Chris and my adorable twin granddaughters. Who make me realise how fortunate I am to have a family! That includes my close friends, family, cousins and nieces who have showed me so much love and support.

And to those searching for the truth about their own past . . . never give up hope. I didn't!